Fast Metabolism Weight Loss Diet Plan

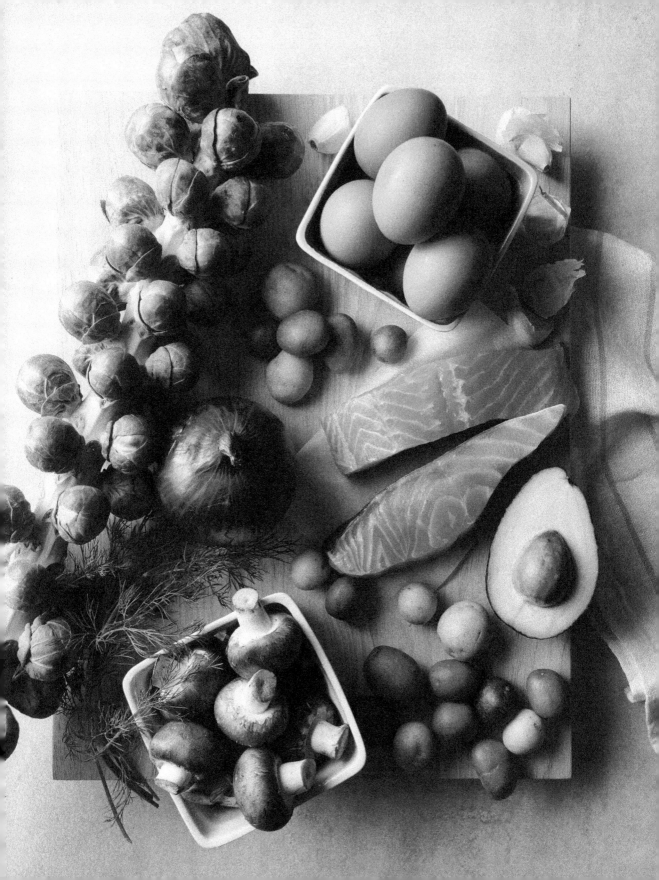

FAST METABOLISM
WEIGHT LOSS
DIET PLAN

RESET HEALTH AND ACHIEVE LASTING WEIGHT LOSS

Megan Johnson McCullough, MA

ROCKRIDGE
PRESS

For general information on our other products and services or to obtain technical support, please contact our Customer Care Department within the United States at (866) 744-2665, or outside the United States at (510) 253-0500.

Rockridge Press publishes its books in a variety of electronic and print formats. Some content that appears in print may not be available in electronic books, and vice versa.

TRADEMARKS: Rockridge Press and the Rockridge Press logo are trademarks or registered trademarks of Callisto Media Inc. and/or its affiliates, in the United States and other countries, and may not be used without written permission. All other trademarks are the property of their respective owners. Rockridge Press is not associated with any product or vendor mentioned in this book.

Interior and Cover Designer: Brian Lewis
Art Producer: Samantha Ulban
Editor: Annie Choi

Photography © 2021 Marija Vidal, cover and p.ii; Nadine Greeff, p.vi-vii; Hélène Dujardin, pp.iix, 2, 42, 44, 62; Andrew Purcell, p.18; Jennifer Davick, p.82; Darren Muir pp.104-105; Annabelle Breakley, p.120. Food Styling by Victoria Woollard, cover. Author Photo Courtesy of JP Casiano.

ISBN: Print 978-1-64876-314-4 | eBook 978-1-64876-315-1

R0

Cover recipe: Green Smoothie Bowl, page 50

This book is dedicated to my husband, Carl McCullough, who has loved me and accepted me at every size and shape I've ever been.

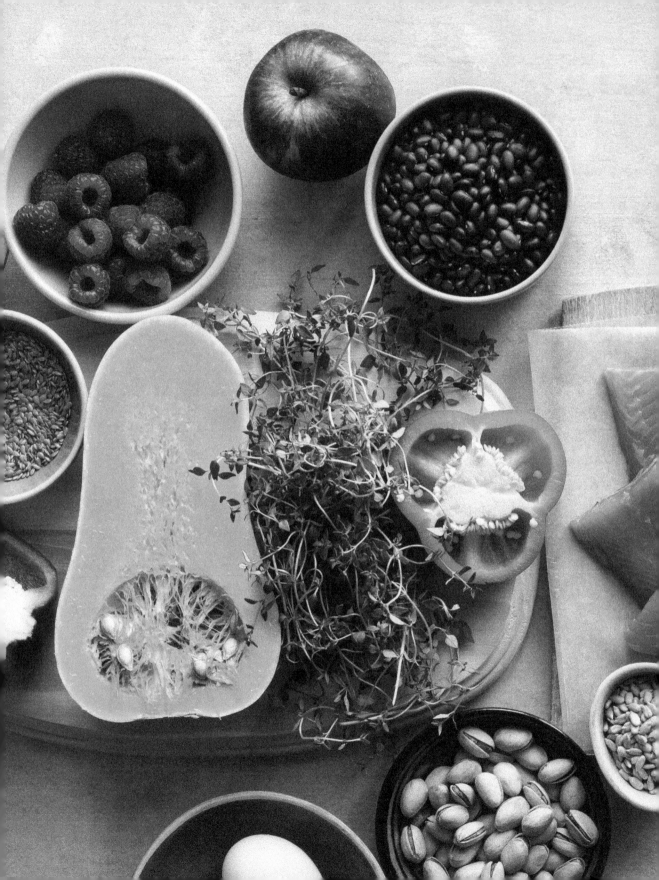

CONTENTS

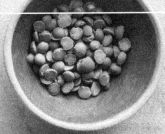

Introduction

I'm Megan Johnson McCullough, MA, and I am happy to share this fast metabolism plan with you. As the owner of Every BODY's Fit fitness studio in Oceanside, California, a professional natural bodybuilder, an NASM Master Trainer, a published author, and a candidate for my doctorate in health and human performance, my mission is to help every BODY become the best version of themselves.

If you've struggled to lose weight like I have, you know that those digits on the scale can trigger an ugly war between your mind and body. Persistent weight gain can wreak havoc on body image and self-esteem, not to mention the negative health factors associated with being overweight. We want to gain control over our weight and lose pounds. Losing weight is hard, but when your metabolism is out of balance, it can be even harder.

I'm a professional natural bodybuilder, ranked second in the world, but it took years for me to take control of my metabolism and eating habits. As a fitness trainer and fitness model, I looked fit on the outside, but I was no stranger to overeating behind closed doors. After a knee surgery from a basketball injury in college, I gained more than 50 pounds. I turned to food to suppress feeling homesick and not being able to play my sport. I may have binged on "healthier" choices, but a gallon of almond milk with a box of whole-grain cereal as one meal will put the pounds on.

Based on my own experience with weight loss, I focus on meal prep and taking my designated amounts of food to work with me to have more control over my diet. My approach is to first focus on what I'm eating, then focus on how much I'm eating, and then prepare each week in advance to keep this eating schedule. The scale is not the only indication of progress, either. Take "before" photos and use a pair of jeans as your circumference baseline to see how they fit after five weeks. Your organs, joints, and muscles will be so happy you decided to follow this plan.

This book will provide everything you need to know about jump-starting your metabolism in five steps, including a 5-week meal plan to help you reboot and maintain a healthy metabolism. The recipes have been developed to make you feel full as you shed the weight and lose the fat. Exercise will also be a key component of this plan. I'll put you to work so that your metabolism will start to work for you. I only wish I had that nutritional education in my younger years.

After five weeks, you will begin to see weight loss as the result of boosting your metabolism. But this isn't a race that ends after five weeks. To keep these results, you will need to transition into a maintenance phase that is sustainable, and I will also teach you how to do this. As you put the plan into action, your metabolism will be given the green light to work more efficiently. I wish you well with all the happiness and health your body deserves. Let's get started!

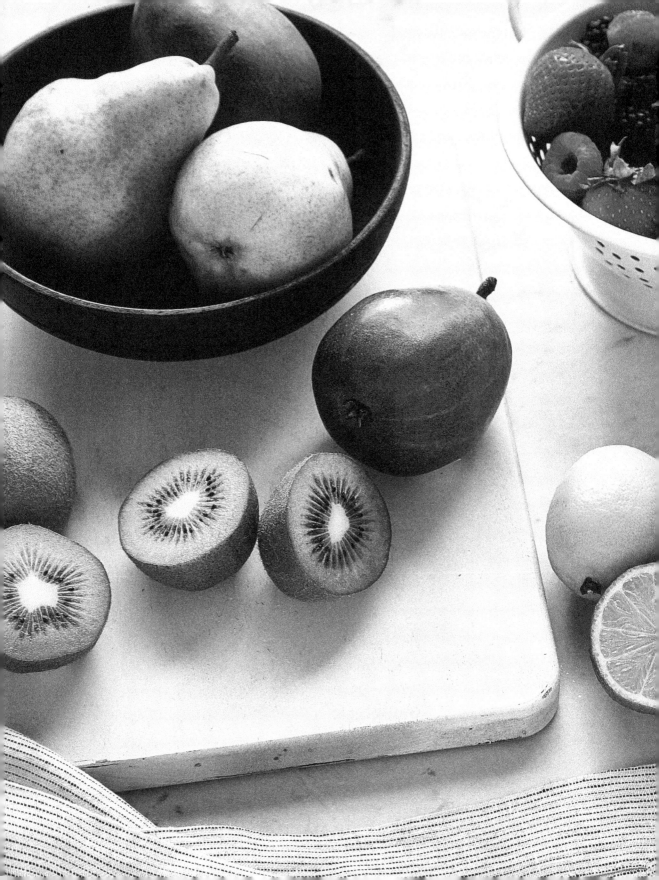

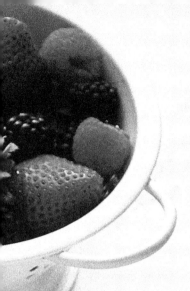

PART
01

JUMP-STARTING YOUR HEALTH

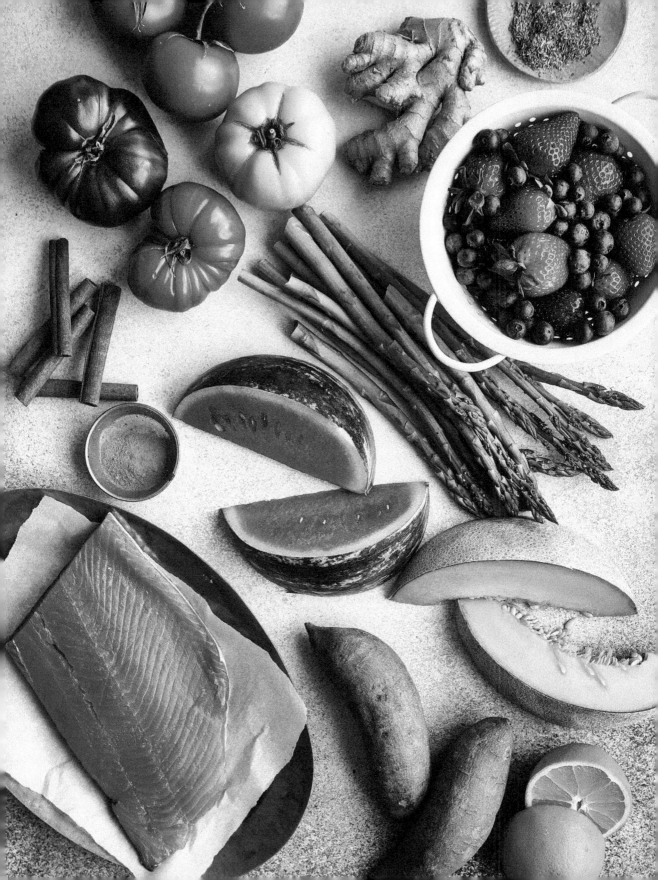

CHAPTER 1

METABOLISM AND WEIGHT LOSS

Let me guess, you have tried dieting before. Even if you were successful, you may have found yourself in the same predicament once again . . . frustrated with weight that you can't seem to shed. This time, you can get out of the diet cycle and take back control of your weight loss. In this chapter, you will learn how your metabolism works so you can understand the underlying factors that could be affecting your weight. Then I'll show you how to jump-start your metabolism so you can shed those pounds once and for all. Over the next five weeks, your metabolism is going to become a construction zone. Your health is the most important project you can work on. The tools are being given to you.

Making Sense of Metabolism

Metabolism is the process of your body converting what you eat and drink into the energy necessary for all functions (breathing, blood circulation, repairing cells, etc.). The calories in food and drinks combine with oxygen to release this energy. The number of calories a person needs per day to perform these functions is called your basal metabolic rate (BMR). This is the baseline number your body needs to consume to live. This means that consuming more or less than your BMR affects your body weight.

BMR is uniquely individualized because it takes into account a person's body size and body composition. Individuals who are larger or even those who have more muscle burn more calories in general, even when resting. Your age also matters, because as we age, muscle mass decreases while fat increases, which leads to fewer calories being burned. In general, men burn more calories than women, making gender another factor in metabolic rate. Compared to women of the same age and height, men generally have more muscle and less fat. Your metabolic rate also depends on how much physical activity you do.

Gaining weight is actually quite complicated and isn't just about eating too many calories. It can be influenced by a number of factors, including genetics, diet, hormones, stress, sleep, medications, lifestyle, and activity levels. The good news is that you can control some of these factors by changing your diet, minimizing stress, getting enough sleep, and being physically active. When you take charge of what you can control, you can help boost your metabolism and make it work efficiently for you.

Metabolism is related to how many calories your body needs. The food we consume can be converted into energy, get excreted, or be stored. If we take in more calories than we can burn or excrete, they will get stored, often as fat.

Weight gain is also due to the role of insulin. After you eat, especially if you had a high-carbohydrate or sugar-filled meal, your blood glucose level rises. This makes the pancreas secrete more insulin. Insulin tells the muscles and the other organs in the body to use the glucose for energy, but it also tells the fat cells to store fat to be used later. This accumulation of fat continues because the other cells burn glucose (not fat) for energy. Glucose comes from starches, sugars, and grains, so the more easily digestible (simple) these foods are, the more quickly they spike insulin levels. In just a short period of time after the spike, your blood sugar will quickly drop, leaving you feeling hungry and with less energy. Frequent insulin spikes can confuse your metabolism and lead to long-term negative health concerns. Foods rich in fiber slow down this insulin spike, so fiber-filled options will become our friends.

In order to lose weight, you need to have a calorie deficit. This could be achieved by eating fewer calories or by burning more calories than you eat ("calories in and calories out"). Counting calories is not always the magic trick to lose weight but is one way to offset weight gain. Taking control of your metabolism (getting it to speed up) means taking control of what you *can* control and understanding what you *cannot*. Play to your body's strengths and don't let the weaknesses discourage you. Some people do seem to lose weight faster than others, but focus on *your* body. Your hormones, genetic makeup, and body composition are unique, so even if you eat the same food and perform the same activities as someone else, that does not mean your body will respond (metabolize) the same way. It is not fair to yourself to compare how you lose weight to how someone else does. Their body has different caloric needs. You clean up your home, car, and workplace, and now you are going to clean up your eating.

FIVE STEPS TO RESET

Focusing on what you can control to meet *your* body's needs is critical. Although we would all like a magic trick that makes the weight disappear, there is not a one-size-fits-all magic formula for speeding up metabolism. However, there are key things you can do to positively impact your metabolism and aid in weight loss. These controllable factors are completely in your power to practice daily. In the rest of this chapter, we are going to focus on the following:

1. Love Your Organs

2. Follow an Anti-Inflammatory Diet

3. Know Your Timing

4. Build Your Muscles

5. Practice Good Habits

Step 1: Love Your Organs

Our bodies are designed like machines with many parts working together every single second of our lives. There are vital organs in our bodies that we must keep functioning efficiently to stay healthy. These core organs include the brain, heart, kidney, liver, skin, pancreas, lungs, small intestine, large intestine, and stomach. The best way to help the body do what it's built to do is by choosing foods that aid and repair these organs while reducing our exposure to environmental toxins. Leafy green vegetables, nuts, seeds, berries, poultry, fish such as salmon, and sweet potatoes are all examples of clean foods that are packed with nutrients that repair our organs. These are "productive" calories that go to work for us.

On the other hand, foods loaded with grease, fat, and artificial chemicals make the body work harder because these are "empty" calories that are toxic to the digestive system and cells. Habits such as smoking cigarettes make the lungs work harder, taking multiple medications due to poor health makes the liver work harder, and the accumulation of excess fat makes the heart's job much more difficult. Think of the qualities you look for in a good boss. Wouldn't you want someone in charge to add positivity and good decision-making to your day versus someone who is negative and adds toxicity? Recognize yourself as the boss of *your* body and metabolism. All the organs are bound to be more productive when they favor the person in charge. But when your organs aren't healthy, they will communicate and demonstrate this through deteriorating health.

In terms of your metabolism, it is important to pay particular attention to your liver. The liver is where carbohydrates, fat, and amino acids (proteins) are metabolized. You do not want to eat foods that will disrupt the liver's job. Foods high in fats and foreign chemicals make the liver work harder to break down these substances, adding more time and stress to its job. This is because the liver produces carnitine, which influences about 90 percent of your metabolism. The faster your body produces this carnitine in the liver, the faster your metabolism is. Therefore, you should let all your organs feel loved, but it's especially important to pamper your liver when you want to boost your metabolism.

REDUCING YOUR TOXIC LOAD

We encounter many different toxins on a daily basis, and sometimes because they are so common and found in so many items, we underestimate the toll they can take on our metabolic functioning. Toxins are found in many of the foods we eat in the form of pesticides, herbicides, and synthetic hormones found in meats or genetically modified foods. These toxins aren't limited to our foods and can be found even in skin-care products, makeup, the air we breathe, and many types of prescription drugs. Many scented items, like candles, cleaning products, air fresheners, and lotions, can be filled with toxins.

The problem is that many of these toxins that we are repeatedly exposed to act like estrogen in the body, which could even cause girls to enter puberty early. Our natural testosterone levels can become overwhelmed by this fake estrogen. Excess estrogen can also raise insulin sensitivity. This hormonal imbalance can lead to weight gain.

What you can do to help minimize exposure is to eat as much organic food as possible, with a focus on fresh produce and lean meats. Choose fewer processed and packaged items. This helps lessen the artificial ingredients, added sugar, and processed simple carbohydrates that you consume. Eating clean takes on a whole new importance when you know it can affect your metabolism.

Step 2: Follow an Anti-Inflammatory Diet

The dietary approach of this book is going to focus on eating anti-inflammatory foods, which means lots of fruits and vegetables, plant-based proteins, fresh herbs and spices, and healthy fatty fish. Foods that are processed, overcooked, or greasy are not good choices, because they can quickly spike insulin levels and become stored as fat. Quick-to-digest foods equate to quick spikes in blood sugar. It's time to eat more naturally, which helps your metabolism work with you rather than in a constant fight for you. More specifically, this book will emphasize the following:

Focus on Whole Foods

This is the simple idea of eating the way our ancestors did more than 100 years ago. Whole foods are those that are as close to their natural form as possible. They have not been through industrial production lines, packaged, preserved for shelf life, colored, or loaded with artificial ingredients. Think of this as having a chicken breast versus chicken nuggets.

Avoid Sugar, Dairy, and Gluten

Your stomach and digestive system have feelings, too, meaning they're sensitive to what you consume. Sugar is everywhere and highly addictive. It rots our teeth and our health. Food manufacturers know this and play on the fact that sugar triggers the brain's reward system. Like a drug, sugar makes us want more and more of it, but it can lead to weight gain and metabolic disorders like diabetes.

We all grew up with the notion that drinking milk was necessary for strong bones. However, after young childhood, somewhere between two and five, our bodies stop producing lactase in the same amount. This is the digestive enzyme needed to break down dairy. Realistically, we humans are the only species that drinks milk from another species, and our bodies just aren't designed to digest dairy efficiently, which can add to weight gain. Avoid dairy when you can.

When you think of the word "gluten," think about the term "glue." Gluten is a sticky protein found in wheat, barley, and rye. Its ability to form a stretchy structure is what gives bread its shape and size. The very same thing happens in your stomach. Gluten can make you feel bloated and uncomfortable and that is why bread, pizza crust, bagels, and pastries can make you feel full, but only for a short time. Many gluten-containing foods are refined carbs that spike insulin. You quickly digest them and then crave them once again in a short period. If you know you tolerate gluten well, choose whole-grain options.

Eat Mostly Plants

This doesn't mean becoming a vegetarian or a vegan. It simply means eating the types of foods that offer our bodies the necessary nutrients, vitamins, minerals, carbohydrates, proteins, and fats for optimal health. A mostly plant-based diet will help maintain a healthy weight.

Choose Healthy Fats

Eat heart-healthy fats, not those that clog the arteries. Healthy fats come from avocados, nuts, olive oil, and fish like salmon that contain omega-3 fatty acids.

Choose Carbs Wisely

Complex carbs such as sweet potatoes have more fiber than simple carbs like white bread that only make us feel full for a short period of time. Simple carbs spike our blood sugar, making us feel good, but the crash and burn will come.

Satiation Is Key

Whole foods are loaded with fiber, so you will feel full and satisfied, not deprived. Eating lean protein also makes you feel fuller longer and more energized.

RESETTING ON THE PLAN

Your palate has been confused by toxins and tastebud-pleasing choices that have equated food to a rewarding drug rather than a nutritious necessity. Your brain has been telling your metabolism that it needs more foods with sugar and starches. Before starting on the plan, you will need to recalibrate your palate.

This will involve drastically reducing all sugars and starches for the first four days and then slowly reintroducing them. These may include even natural foods like fruit and high-starch vegetables, because the brain recognizes any form of sugar—processed or natural—as sugar and responds in the same way. Although your body digests the sugar in fruit more slowly, the temptation for table sugar can still exist. Starches such as those found in white potatoes still break down into glucose (sugar).

You will bring these foods back, but you have to start at ground zero to give your metabolism the best environment to speed up. Look for labels like "sugar-free" and "grain-free" for elimination-friendly recipes. In this book, "sugar-free" will mean no added sugars in the form of table sugar or processed sugars.

FOODS TO ENJOY

VEGETABLES (FRESH, FROZEN, OR CANNED WITHOUT ADDED SODIUM)

Alliums
Chives
Garlic*
Leeks
Onions*
Scallions
Shallots

Cruciferous Vegetables*
Arugula
Bok choy
Broccoli
Brussels sprouts
Cabbage
Cauliflower
Collard greens
Kale
Kohlrabi
Mizuna
Mustard greens
Radish greens
Romanesco broccoli/
Roman cauliflower
Turnip greens

Dark Green Leafy Vegetables
Lettuces, especially
romaine*
Spinach*
Swiss chard*

Root Vegetables
Beets
Carrots
Celery root/celeriac
Radishes
Rutabagas
Sweet potatoes
Turnips
Winter squash

Other Vegetables
Asparagus
Bell peppers
Corn
Fermented, probiotic
vegetables*
Green beans
Mushrooms

FRUIT (FRESH, FROZEN, OR CANNED WITHOUT ADDED SUGAR)

Apples
Apricots
Avocados
Bananas
Berries*
Citrus*
Cranberries

Figs
Grapes
Kiwi
Mangos
Melons
Pineapple*
Stone fruit

FATS AND OILS

Nut oils
Olive oil*

Seed oils

WHOLE AND ANCIENT GRAINS

Amaranth*
Brown rice
Buckwheat*
Millet*

Oatmeal*
Popcorn
Quinoa*
Teff*

SEEDS

Chia
Flaxseed*
Hemp
Mustard

Poppy
Pumpkin
Sesame
Sunflower

HERBS AND SPICES

Basil
Bay leaf
Cilantro
Cinnamon*
Clove
Dill
Ginger*
Mint
Nutmeg
Oregano*

Paprika
Parsley
Pepper
Rosemary*
Saffron*
Sage
Tarragon
Thyme
Turmeric*

PROTEINS

Beans*
Tempeh*

Tofu

OTHER

Unsweetened coffee

Unsweetened black
or green tea*

Note: Asterisks indicate foods that are particularly beneficial anti-inflammatory superstars.

CONSIDER WITH CARE

FATS AND OILS

Coconut	Sesame
Corn	Soy
Safflower	Sunflower

WHOLE AND ANCIENT GRAINS

Barley	Spelt
Emmer	Wheat berries
Farro	Whole-grain breads, bulgur, couscous, pastas
Rye	

NUTS AND SEEDS

Peanuts	Tree nuts* (e.g., almonds, cashews, macadamias, pistachios, walnuts*)

DAIRY

Fermented, probiotic dairy* (e.g., kefir, yogurt)	Low-fat and nonfat dairy products (e.g., cheese, milk)

PROTEINS

Eggs	Poultry (skinless white meat)
Fish* (e.g., cod, flounder, halibut, mackerel, salmon,* sardines,* tuna)	Shellfish (e.g., mussels, oysters, scallops)
Pork (very lean cuts, such as pork tenderloin)	Soy (e.g., edamame/ soybeans, tofu, tempeh)

OTHER

Dark chocolate	Red wine

AVOID

FATS AND OILS

Butter	Margarine
Lard	

GRAINS

All refined grains (e.g., white bread and rolls, white pasta, white rice)	Packaged, processed grain-based snacks and desserts (e.g., biscuits, cakes, cereals, cookies, crackers, muffins)
	Pastries

OTHER

Bacon	High-sodium foods
Beef (especially high-fat cuts, beef charred on the grill, and corn-fed beef—typically any that is not grass-fed)	Packaged and processed foods
	Packaged, processed meat alternatives (e.g., "garden burgers," faux chicken)
Full-fat dairy (e.g., butter, cheese, cream, half-and-half, ice cream)	Refined added sugars (brown sugar, confectioners' sugar, high-fructose corn syrup, white sugar)
High-fat foods (especially those with high saturated fats or trans fats)	

Step 3: Know Your Timing

When you eat affects your metabolism. In fact, irregular eating can increase the risks of obesity, high blood pressure, high cholesterol, and high blood sugar. Consistency is key, especially as you are training your metabolism. When your body knows what to expect and when, it will start to trust your decision making and start to improve its performance for you. Proper nutrition requires proper calories at the times your body needs them. Nutrient timing doesn't involve gulping down a protein shake after a workout or rushing through meals. The body has windows of opportunity throughout the day when it is in ideal condition to absorb nutrients.

Limiting calories to certain times of the day helps avoid excess calories, which in turn can cut calories and lead to weight loss. You are setting a schedule for your metabolism that will entail three meals and one snack per day. When your body knows replenishment is around the corner, it will not hold on to calories and fat to be stored when needed. It will decide to convert them to energy to be used, because it knows the tank will be refilled. If your metabolism can't depend on you to help it out and take care of it, why should it trust you and work faster only to feel empty and depleted later?

The correct timing of eating has been shown to increase weight loss, improve blood sugar control, and increase longevity. Even brain function has been shown to improve. Your individual needs for eating times will depend on your responsibilities, commitments, sleeping hours, activity level, and use of certain medications. For example, if you know you have to take a medication on an empty stomach and it must be first thing in the morning, you need to coordinate your food timing appropriately. In this case you could wake up, take your medication, then start the timing of your eating 30 minutes later. Before reading this book, you might have skipped breakfast and then ravenously eaten at lunchtime, but this needs to be fixed. Timing is everything, and this time your metabolism is going to thank you.

INTERMITTENT FASTING 101

The practice of fasting has been around for thousands of years. Intermittent fasting is a cycle of eating targeted to lose weight and burn fat. This book will address the 16/8 method, a popular choice for beginners that is easy to follow. Because it is less restrictive and more flexible than other fasting methods, it is easier to fit into your lifestyle. In this method, you consume calorie-containing foods and beverages during a set window of 8 hours per day while abstaining from them during the other 16 hours. This helps your metabolism by improving blood sugar control.

Anyone can be a good candidate for the 16/8 method, provided that the 8-hour window is sustainable and can be followed consistently. Examples of this approach would be eating between the hours of 12 p.m. and 8 p.m. and fasting overnight for the remaining 16 hours or eating between the hours of 9 a.m. and 5 p.m. and fasting for the rest. You can drink calorie-free beverages such as water and tea during the fast to help. It is very important to avoid bingeing or eating junk food when you break the fast. If the fasting period becomes a burden, you may need to adjust those hours. If you take medications, these should be considered for timing.

Step 4: Build Your Muscles

If ever there was a reason to start building muscles, now's the time. Fact: Muscle mass and muscle tissue burn more calories even at rest compared to fat. Who doesn't want to burn calories while sleeping or watching TV? This doesn't mean you have to channel your inner bodybuilder. Simple weight-bearing exercises can go a long way in changing your metabolism. Ladies, don't be scared of weights adding too much muscle, because a typical female body does not contain enough testosterone to bulk up quickly.

Unlike the timing of eating, exercise is more about getting it done rather than when you get it done. Any time of day works so long as the exercise gets done. Even doing 10-minute segments throughout the day is far more beneficial than skipping days and sitting. Ideally, resistance training three to five days per week can help rev up your metabolism. How long your sessions should last depends on what activity you are doing and at what intensity.

Cardio is a great heart-healthy exercise that can complement weight-bearing activities. But too much cardio can lead to burning through muscle, so a good alternative to is to raise your heart rate during resistance training activities. Pounding the treadmill or elliptical won't change your body the way weight training will, but it is still good for your heart. A solid effort for 30 to 60 minutes is a good baseline to aspire to that will include both a cardiovascular activity and a resistance training component. Here are the exercises I recommend for improving metabolism:

HIIT (High Intensity Interval Training)

High intensity interval training (HIIT) involves intervals of high-level effort and active recovery periods. HIIT is great for boosting metabolism because the cardiovascular system is challenged by the changing levels of heart rate.

For example, using light dumbbells to build muscle, perform 20 seconds of jumping jacks followed by 10 seconds of a light jog or march in place. Repeating this pattern 10 times will total 5 minutes. Follow this pattern using those same light dumbbells to perform ice skaters, burpees, punches, jump squats, and alternating high knees to opposite elbow. This is 30 minutes of work, and all you need is a little space, a couple of dumbbells, and your body.

Strength Training

In general, to increase strength, resistance training will involve three to five sets of 10 to 12 repetitions of each exercise. You want to use weights that challenge you so that by the fourth or fifth set you are no longer able to repeat that exercise. You could target different parts of the body on different workout days.

For example, one day you could focus on bicep and tricep movements while another day you focus on glutes and hamstrings (legs). These exercises can be done with free weights or machines. If you don't have access to these, you can use your own body weight.

Stretching and Resting

It is important to allow your body to recover from exercise so that it can experience hypertrophy (muscle growth). When fatigued or overstressed, your muscles will not efficiently perform movement patterns. This can lead to injury, and exercising when fatigued won't maximize the quality of the workout you want to achieve. Stretch either statically, actively, or using tools such as a foam roller to help blood flow reach these worked areas. One way to rest and recover efficiently is by not working the same muscles during successive workouts within a 24-hour period. This way, you can still burn fat and calories but not add stress to previously targeted body parts.

Step 5: Practice Good Habits

Lifestyle factors beyond diet and exercise also affect metabolism. Recognizing the strengths and areas for improvement in your daily habits is important for success.

Incorporating Mindfulness

Whenever you can, slow down when eating. When we are rushed and distracted, we tend to eat more, and it becomes harder to tune in to our hunger cues. Try chewing more slowly, which will allow your food to reach your stomach in stages versus all at once. Think of the rule for washing your hands, taking the time to thoroughly chew for 20 seconds. This engages your hunger signals sooner and can help you eat less.

Recognizing you are full requires you to eat with just the food in front of you, not while watching TV, reading, typing, or texting. Tune in to the food so that you don't keep eating mindlessly. Know that it is okay to feel hungry, but keep in mind that hunger doesn't always mean you need to have an entire meal. For example, when you feel hungry, drink water first, and if you're still hungry, a quality snack like carrots or apples from the Foods to Enjoy table (page 10) can do the trick.

Managing Stress

Chronic stress can cause your cortisol levels to rise. When they do, they are the devil of hunger signals telling you that you need food to suppress your emotions. You can feel the emotion, but that doesn't mean you have to eat it. The timing of your eating will be taunted by a desire for the wrong food choices at the wrong time. Your body starts to crave unnecessary carbohydrates when you are stressed, and the resulting imbalance of hormones will affect your metabolism.

Sleeping Well

Getting regular and enough sleep is another habit the metabolism appreciates. At least seven hours of sleep is a good baseline to let your body rest. When you don't get adequate sleep, your body produces more ghrelin (a hormone that signals hunger) and less leptin (a hormone that signals you are full). Poor sleep can increase your appetite, which interferes with your ability to fast. It also does not allow your body the recovery time necessary to build muscle and maintain the weight you want.

TIPS FOR SUCCESS

You already have what it takes to succeed on this plan, but here are some tips to help set you up for success:

Timing: Although the perfect time won't ever arise, pick a time that allows you to make this plan a priority (not during the holidays or when work is busiest).

Prep: Use the weekly Prep Ahead advice at the end of each shopping list to plan and make food ahead and stay organized. As with anything in life, good time management makes this all possible. Act like your own personal assistant.

Track your progress: Take "before" pictures, keep a food and activity log, and even keep a journal of your daily accomplishments and feelings.

Stay hydrated: Water is your body's necessary lubricant to make all operations possible. It can also make you feel fuller. Water is also needed for digestion and recovery. Keep a bottle close at hand at all times.

Don't compare: Your progress is unique to *you* and your plan. Don't pay attention to what the person next to you is doing.

Mistakes happen: Minor slipups or even major ones don't mean you have to stop this plan. Fix it, pivot, and get right back on track.

Maintaining Health in the Long Run

The first one to two weeks of this plan will serve as the foundation to jump-start your metabolism while helping you take control of your weight. Once you get to week 5 in the meal plan, which is how I recommend you eat most of the time, you may notice that it's quite doable. You will see that it can fit into your lifestyle. Review and keep the week 5 plan in mind as an example of how to eat to help you maintain your weight loss over time.

Reintroducing certain foods will require portion control and paying attention to your hunger cues. When adding back treats or other foods you don't want to give up forever, try eating just two bites and leaving it alone. Telling yourself something is not allowed can sometimes lead to more cravings. When you let your body know that you can have a cookie every now and then, you won't feel deprived or lacking. This meal plan is a tool that you can revisit when needed, say if you gain 10 pounds after a surgery or after a particularly stressful period at work. Life happens, but now you have a plan that takes only five weeks of your life to produce results. With this fast metabolism boost, you can take charge of your metabolism.

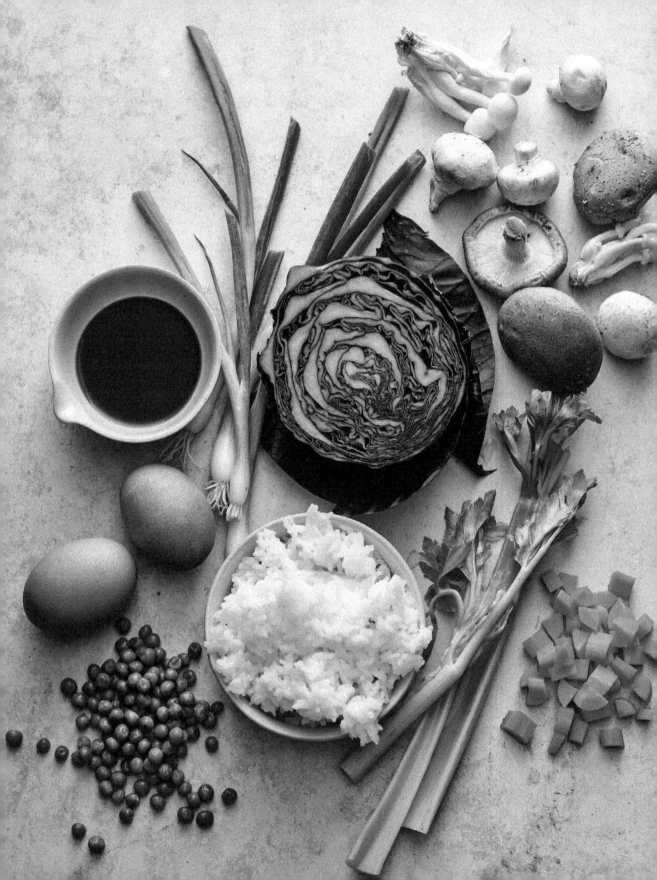

CHAPTER 2

YOUR 5-WEEK MEAL PLAN

This 5-week plan will provide you with the guidance necessary to eat three meals and one healthy snack per day. This eating period will take place during your self-designated eight hours of the 16/8 method (see page 13). You will be given a shopping list to make recipes suitable for this plan that will retrain and direct your metabolism to kick itself into gear. Exercise is encouraged and explained as well.

About the Plan

This plan is designed for one person and will include three meals and one healthy snack per day. You still have your life to live with all its demands, so the idea is to make eating clean as easy as possible. The plan focuses on quick recipes that yield nutritious and delicious foods. It offers plenty of make-ahead tips for the weekend before. Leftovers will be a go-to strategy as well.

The first week of the plan is set up to detox your system by eliminating certain foods and to introduce the dietary principles that will propel your metabolism, as explained in chapter 1. As the weeks progress, the plan will reintroduce foods eliminated in the first week. The final week of the plan will represent what I recommend as a typical eating plan to help you maintain your results. See "Maintaining Health in the Long Run" (page 17) for more advice on reintroducing foods and how to incorporate a metabolism diet plan into your lifestyle.

ADDING INTERMITTENT FASTING

Intermittent fasting is a pattern of eating where you cycle fasting and eating. It can be a strategy when you are trying to train your metabolism and set yourself up for time-focused eating.

To incorporate intermittent fasting into your plan, pick eight hours of your day that will allow you to eat every two hours while fasting outside that eight-hour window. For example, you could pick eating from 12 p.m. to 8 p.m., which would mean waking up and not eating for a period of time. Or you could decide to eat from 8 a.m. to 4 p.m. or 9 a.m. to 5 p.m. A popular strategy is to leave the fasting hours for when you are sleeping. Consider when you will be exercising, as well. Having energy from food is necessary. For example, you wouldn't want to stop eating at 3 p.m. and then exercise at 7 p.m. when you might be feeling hungry.

Intermittent fasting needs to be oriented around your personal health situations, especially if you take medications that are affected by food intake. For example, if you know you must take your prescription on an empty stomach, take it during fasting. Or if you know the medication upsets your stomach when it is empty, take it during eating hours.

Exercising on the Plan

If you have not exercised in some time, begin at a light-to-moderate pace, starting with 15 minutes of aerobic activity (walking, jogging, swimming, or biking) followed by 30 minutes of strength training. For strength training, begin with lighter weights, focusing on 15 to 20 repetitions of each exercise for three to five sets. Each week, try adding a few minutes to your cardio time or increasing the intensity level. For the resistance training portion, you can add weight and lessen the number of repetitions.

If you have already been exercising and might be concerned about reducing calories, you may need to add an extra protein shake or complex carbohydrate snack option to meet your energy needs. Be sure to coordinate eating times with exercise times so that you can take advantage of the calories you do eat for fuel during workouts. For example, working out on an empty stomach doesn't necessarily fuel your tank to perform physical activity. As a general rule, try to eat one to two hours before exercise and within one hour after exercise to refuel your body for recovery purposes. You may also have to consider doing less cardio for the five weeks of the plan to offset low caloric intake.

Managing Expectations

This jump-start plan is designed to help you shed pounds quickly. Therefore, expect to lose more weight in the first few weeks than in the final weeks, when you will be reintroducing foods like fruit and starchy vegetables. Transitioning off this plan will require you to continue to exercise and maybe even become more physically active to maintain the effects of "calories in and calories out." You might feel tired or hungry or have low energy at first, but that will be temporary, and each week you will find yourself adjusting.

Your self-esteem and confidence may perk up, and your clothes may start to fit better. But the benefits of this plan are not just external. Your organs will appreciate your efforts. Establishing healthy routines will prove to yourself that you can do this and that you can live your life with more energy and control. Remember, every single form of progress counts, and that could be as simple as looking at yourself in the mirror and smiling because you feel good about taking care of yourself.

5-Week Meal Plan

Before starting each week, check the Prep Ahead (Sunday) tips at the end of each shopping list to see what you can make ahead the weekend before. Recipes in *italics* indicate leftovers from a previous day.

Week 1

	BREAKFAST	LUNCH	DINNER	SNACK
MONDAY	Gingerbread Smoothie (page 47)	Spicy Broccoli and Chicken Slaw (page 72)	Ground Turkey and Cauliflower Rice Stir-Fry (page 94)	2 tablespoons Guacamole (page 110) with ¼ red bell pepper, sliced
TUESDAY	Broccoli and Bell Pepper Frittata Muffins (page 57)	Ginger-Lime Tuna Salad (page 79)	Ginger-Lime Cod Tacos (page 100)	10 blanched almonds
WEDNESDAY	*Gingerbread Smoothie*	*Spicy Broccoli and Chicken Slaw*	*Ground Turkey and Cauliflower Rice Stir-Fry*	1 cup Kale Chips (page 113)
THURSDAY	*Broccoli and Bell Pepper Frittata Muffins*	*Ginger-Lime Tuna Salad*	*Ginger-Lime Cod Tacos*	*2 tablespoons Guacamole with ¼ red bell pepper, sliced*
FRIDAY	Pumpkin Spice Smoothie (page 46)	*Spicy Broccoli and Chicken Slaw*	Baked Cod with Lemon and Scallions (page 101)	10 blanched almonds
SATURDAY	*Broccoli and Bell Pepper Frittata Muffins*	Chicken Meatball Pho (page 74)	Cod Piccata with Zoodles (page 98)	*1 cup Kale Chips*
SUNDAY	*Pumpkin Spice Smoothie*	Southwestern Shrimp and Avocado Salad (page 81)	Hand-Cut Zoodles with Turkey Bolognese (page 95)	1 hard-boiled egg

Shopping List

PRODUCE

- ☐ Avocados (2)
- ☐ Bell pepper, any color (1)
- ☐ Bell peppers, red (3)
- ☐ Broccoli (2 large bunches)
- ☐ Broccoli slaw, 1 (9-ounce) bag
- ☐ Carrots (2)
- ☐ Cauliflower rice (4 cups)
- ☐ Cilantro (4 bunches)
- ☐ Coleslaw mix or shredded cabbage, 2 (9-ounce) bags
- ☐ Garlic (3 heads)
- ☐ Ginger (1 large piece)
- ☐ Greens, mixed, 1 (9-ounce) bag
- ☐ Jalapeño (1)
- ☐ Kale (1 bunch)
- ☐ Lemons (5)
- ☐ Lettuce, butter (1 head)
- ☐ Limes (8)
- ☐ Onion, red (1)
- ☐ Onion, yellow (1)
- ☐ Oranges (2)
- ☐ Parsley (1 bunch)
- ☐ Scallions (4 bunches)
- ☐ Shallots (3)
- ☐ Thyme (1 bunch)
- ☐ Tomatoes, cherry (1 pint)
- ☐ Zucchini, medium (10)

PROTEIN: MEAT, POULTRY, AND SEAFOOD

- ☐ Chicken, 1 pound boneless, skinless breasts
- ☐ Chicken, ground (1 pound)
- ☐ Cod (1 pound)
- ☐ Cod, 8 (4-ounce) fillets
- ☐ Eggs (2 dozen)
- ☐ Shrimp, baby, cooked (6 ounces)
- ☐ Tuna, water-packed, 2 (3-ounce) cans or pouches
- ☐ Turkey breast, ground (2 pounds)

DAIRY

- ☐ Milk, nondairy, plain (1 quart)
- ☐ Yogurt, nonfat, plain (8 ounces)

CONDIMENTS, HERBS, SPICES, AND OILS

- ☐ Avocado oil
- ☐ Chinese hot mustard powder
- ☐ Cinnamon
- ☐ Cloves, ground
- ☐ Fish sauce
- ☐ Garlic powder
- ☐ Ginger, ground
- ☐ Herbal tea, ginger, 1 bag
- ☐ Hot sauce, sugar-free
- ☐ Italian seasoning, dried
- ☐ Molasses, blackstrap
- ☐ Mustard, Dijon
- ☐ Nutmeg, ground
- ☐ Red chili flakes
- ☐ Sesame oil
- ☐ Soy sauce, reduced-sodium
- ☐ Star anise (1)
- ☐ Stevia
- ☐ Tahini
- ☐ Vanilla extract

NUTS AND SEEDS

- ☐ Almonds, blanched
- ☐ Sesame seeds

CANNED, PACKAGED, AND PANTRY STAPLES

- ☐ Almond flour
- ☐ Broth, vegetable, low-sodium (48 ounces)
- ☐ Capers
- ☐ Pumpkin puree, unsweetened, 1 (14-ounce) can
- ☐ Tomatoes, crushed, 1 (28-ounce) can
- ☐ Water chestnuts, 1 (4-ounce) can

SHOPPING TIPS

☐ For the pantry staples, you may only need to buy some of them this week and they'll last. Double-check your pantry before you shop to make sure you have everything you need.

☐ If you plan to make your own broth, you'll need to purchase vegetables for broth and omit the premade broth.

PREP AHEAD (SUNDAY)

☐ Make the Broccoli and Bell Pepper Frittata Muffins and refrigerate or freeze them in single servings.

☐ Make the chicken for the Spicy Broccoli and Chicken Slaw.

☐ Prep the Ginger-Lime Marinade for the Ground Turkey and Cauliflower Rice Stir-Fry and the Ginger-Lime Tuna Salad and refrigerate it.

☐ Prep the Cilantro-Lime Dressing for the Spicy Broccoli and Chicken Slaw and the Ginger-Lime Cod Tacos and refrigerate it.

☐ Make the broth for the week.

☐ Make the raw cauliflower rice for the Ground Turkey and Cauliflower Rice Stir-Fry.

☐ Make the Guacamole and refrigerate it with plastic wrap pressed onto the surface of the guacamole to prevent oxidation.

☐ Cut the red bell peppers for the guacamole snack.

☐ Hard-boil the eggs for the egg snack.

PREP AHEAD (WEDNESDAY)

☐ Cut the zoodles for the Chicken Meatball Pho, the Cod Piccata with Zoodles, and the Hand-Cut Zoodles with Turkey Bolognese.

☐ Bake the Kale Chips.

Week 2

	BREAKFAST	LUNCH	DINNER	SNACK
MONDAY	Cocoa Chia Smoothie (page 48)	Chicken and Black Bean Salad Lettuce Cups (page 73)	Shrimp Scampi (page 103)	¼ cup plain nonfat yogurt or nondairy yogurt plus ¼ cup blueberries
TUESDAY	Golden Milk Chia Breakfast Pudding with Blueberries (page 51)	Salmon Salad Lettuce Wraps (page 77)	Black Bean Chili (page 85)	1 hard-boiled egg
WEDNES-DAY	*Cocoa Chia Smoothie*	*Chicken and Black Bean Salad Lettuce Cups*	*Shrimp Scampi*	2 tablespoons Hummus (page 108) plus ¼ bell pepper
THURSDAY	*Golden Milk Chia Breakfast Pudding with Blueberries*	*Salmon Salad Lettuce Wraps*	*Black Bean Chili*	1 hard-boiled egg
FRIDAY	Egg and Spinach Scramble (page 59)	*Chicken and Black Bean Salad Lettuce Cups*	Mustard Roasted Pork Tenderloin and Sweet Potatoes (page 96)	*2 tablespoons Hummus plus ¼ bell pepper*
SATURDAY	Turkey Sausage and Sweet Potato Hash (page 61)	Turkey Taco Salad (page 75)	Citrus-Soy Salmon and Veggie Packets (page 97)	¼ cup plain nonfat yogurt or nondairy yogurt plus ¼ cup blueberries
SUNDAY	*Turkey Sausage and Sweet Potato Hash*	Southwestern Shrimp and Avocado Salad (page 81)	Grilled Shrimp with Mango-Cucumber Salsa (page 104)	*2 tablespoons Hummus plus ¼ bell pepper*

Shopping List

PRODUCE

- ☐ Avocado (1)
- ☐ Bell pepper, any color (1)
- ☐ Bell peppers, green (2)
- ☐ Blueberries (1 pint)
- ☐ Chives (1 bunch)
- ☐ Cilantro (3 bunches)
- ☐ Cucumber (1)
- ☐ Dill (1 bunch)
- ☐ Fennel bulb (1)
- ☐ Garlic (2 heads)
- ☐ Greens, mixed, 1 (9-ounce) bag
- ☐ Jalapeños (2)
- ☐ Lemons (5)
- ☐ Lettuce, butter (1 head)
- ☐ Limes (7)
- ☐ Mango (1)
- ☐ Onions, red (2)
- ☐ Onions, yellow (2)
- ☐ Oranges (4)
- ☐ Peas, fresh or frozen (4 ounces)
- ☐ Scallions (1 bunch)
- ☐ Shallots (10)
- ☐ Spinach, baby, 1 (9-ounce) bag
- ☐ Sweet potatoes (6)
- ☐ Tomatoes, large (2)
- ☐ Zucchini, medium (6)

PROTEIN: MEAT, POULTRY, AND SEAFOOD

- ☐ Chicken, 1 pound boneless, skinless breasts
- ☐ Pork, tenderloin (1 pound)
- ☐ Salmon, Pacific, 4 (4-ounce) fillets
- ☐ Salmon, Pacific, 2 (3-ounce) cans
- ☐ Shrimp, baby, cooked (6 ounces)
- ☐ Shrimp, medium (12 ounces)
- ☐ Shrimp, large (1 pound)
- ☐ Turkey breast, ground (1 pound)

DAIRY

- ☐ Milk, nondairy unsweetened, plain (1 quart)
- ☐ Yogurt, nonfat, plain (8 ounces)

NUTS AND SEEDS

- ☐ Chia seeds

CONDIMENTS, HERBS, SPICES, AND OILS

- ☐ Cayenne
- ☐ Chili powder
- ☐ Cloves, ground
- ☐ Cocoa powder, unsweetened
- ☐ Cumin, ground
- ☐ Ginger, ground
- ☐ Honey
- ☐ Maple syrup, pure
- ☐ Olive oil, extra-virgin
- ☐ Oregano, dried
- ☐ Sage, ground
- ☐ Thyme, dried
- ☐ Turmeric, ground
- ☐ Vinegar, apple cider

CANNED, PACKAGED, AND PANTRY STAPLES

- ☐ Black beans, 3 (15-ounce) cans
- ☐ Chickpeas, 1 (15-ounce) can
- ☐ Tomatoes, crushed, 2 (14.5-ounce) cans

SHOPPING TIPS

- Some ingredients will be left over from last week and aren't included in the list.

- For staples, oils, herbs, and spices, you'll probably have these; double-check before shopping to make sure you do—they won't be on shopping lists for recipes carried forward.

PREP AHEAD (SUNDAY)

- Cook the chicken and make the Pico de Gallo and Buttermilk Ranch Dressing for the Chicken and Black Bean Salad Lettuce Cups; refrigerate all.

- Make the Hummus and refrigerate it.

- Make the Black Bean Chili and freeze it in single servings or refrigerate it for up to five days.

- Make the Golden Milk Chia Breakfast Pudding with Blueberries and refrigerate it.

PREP AHEAD (WEDNESDAY)

- Whisk up the Citrus-Soy Marinade for the Citrus-Soy Salmon and Veggie Packets and keep it in the refrigerator until you're ready to use it.

Week 3

	BREAKFAST	LUNCH	DINNER	SNACK
MONDAY	Green Smoothie Bowl (page 50)	Veggie and Hummus Pitas (page 68)	Vegan Pumpkin Soup (page 84)	1 whole Hummus Deviled Egg (page 112) plus ½ cup grapes
TUESDAY	Cranberry-Ginger Oatmeal (page 52)	Beet and Grapefruit Salad (page 64)	Cod Piccata with Zoodles (page 98)	¼ cup blanched almonds
WEDNES-DAY	*Green Smoothie Bowl*	*Beet and Grape-fruit Salad*	*Vegan Pumpkin Soup*	*1 whole Hummus Deviled Egg* plus ½ apple
THURSDAY	*Cranberry-Ginger Oatmeal*	Fiesta Quinoa and Bell Pepper Salad (page 65)	*Cod Piccata with Zoodles*	2 tablespoons almond butter plus ½ apple
FRIDAY	Apple-Cinnamon Overnight Oats (page 53)	*Veggie and Hummus Pitas*	Citrus-Soy Salmon and Veggie Packets (page 97)	¼ cup plain nonfat yogurt plus 2 tablespoons dried cranberries
SATURDAY	Breakfast Burritos (page 58)	Salmon Cobb Salad (page 78)	Ginger-Lime Cod Tacos (page 100)	*1 whole Hummus Deviled Egg*
SUNDAY	Tex-Mex Tofu Scramble (page 60)	Southwestern Shrimp and Avocado Salad (page 81)	Turkey Sloppy Joes (page 91)	¼ cup blanched almonds

Shopping List

PRODUCE

- ☐ Apple, any color (1)
- ☐ Apple, green (1)
- ☐ Avocado (1)
- ☐ Banana (1)
- ☐ Beets (2)
- ☐ Bell pepper, green (1)
- ☐ Bell peppers, red (2)
- ☐ Berries, any kind (1 pint)
- ☐ Chives (1 bunch)
- ☐ Cilantro (2 bunches)
- ☐ Coleslaw mix, 1 (9-ounce) bag
- ☐ Cranberries, dried
- ☐ Dill (1 bunch)
- ☐ Garlic (2 heads)
- ☐ Grapefruit (1)
- ☐ Greens, mixed, 2 (9-ounce) bags
- ☐ Jalapeños (2)
- ☐ Kale (1 bunch)
- ☐ Lemons (4)
- ☐ Limes (6)
- ☐ Onions, red (3)
- ☐ Onions, yellow (2)
- ☐ Orange (1)
- ☐ Parsley (1 bunch)
- ☐ Scallions (2 bunches)
- ☐ Shallots (3)
- ☐ Spinach, baby, 1 (9-ounce) package
- ☐ Tomatoes, cherry (2 pints)
- ☐ Tomatoes, large (4)
- ☐ Zucchini, medium (6)

PROTEIN: MEAT, POULTRY, AND SEAFOOD

- ☐ Chicken, 10 ounces boneless, skinless breasts
- ☐ Cod (1 pound)
- ☐ Cod, 4 (4-ounce) fillets
- ☐ Eggs (1 dozen)

- ☐ Salmon, 4 (4-ounce) fillets
- ☐ Salmon, 1 (6-ounce) fillet
- ☐ Shrimp, baby, cooked (6 ounces)
- ☐ Tofu, silken, extra-firm (6 ounces)
- ☐ Turkey breast, ground (1 pound)

DAIRY

- ☐ Blue cheese crumbles (2 ounces)
- ☐ Milk, nondairy unsweetened, plain
- ☐ Yogurt, nondairy or dairy, plain

NUTS AND SEEDS

- ☐ Almond butter
- ☐ Almonds, blanched
- ☐ Almonds, slivered (2 ounces)
- ☐ Pecans
- ☐ Pepitas
- ☐ Sesame seeds

CONDIMENTS, HERBS, SPICES, AND OILS

- ☐ Cayenne, ground
- ☐ Cinnamon, ground
- ☐ Garlic powder
- ☐ Vinegar, balsamic
- ☐ Worcestershire sauce

BREADS AND GRAINS

- ☐ Hamburger buns, whole wheat (4)
- ☐ Oats, old-fashioned
- ☐ Pita, whole wheat (1 package)
- ☐ Quinoa
- ☐ Tortillas, whole-grain (1 package)

CANNED, PACKAGED, AND PANTRY STAPLES

☐ Black beans,
   1 (14-ounce) can

☐ Black olives, sliced,
   1 (8 ounce) can

☐ Broth, vegetable, low-sodium
   (64 ounces)

☐ Chickpeas, 1 (14-ounce) can

☐ Pumpkin puree, 1 (15-ounce) can

☐ Tomatoes, crushed,
   1 (15-ounce) can

SHOPPING TIPS

☐ Double-check the staples, produce, spices, and dairy lists before you shop, because you may have some left over from last week; replenish as needed.

☐ If you plan to make your own vegetable broth instead of buying it, you'll need to include broth ingredients on your shopping list and omit the canned broth.

PREP AHEAD (SUNDAY)

☐ Roast the beets for the Beet and Grapefruit Salad.

☐ Chop and portion the vegetables for the Veggie and Hummus Pitas.

☐ Cook the quinoa for the Fiesta Quinoa and Bell Pepper Salad and store it in 1-cup servings in the freezer for use throughout the week.

☐ Make the broth if you want to use homemade.

☐ Make the Hummus Deviled Eggs and refrigerate them for up to one week.

PREP AHEAD (WEDNESDAY)

☐ Thaw or make the quinoa, chop the vegetables, and whisk the dressing for the Fiesta Quinoa and Bell Pepper Salad.

Week 4

	BREAKFAST	LUNCH	DINNER	SNACK
MONDAY	Apple-Cinnamon Overnight Oats	Fiesta Quinoa and Bell Pepper Salad	Citrus-Soy Salmon and Veggie Packets (page 97)	Berries with Honeyed Green Tea Yogurt Sauce (page 119)
TUESDAY	Breakfast Burritos	Salmon Cobb Salad	Easy Corn and Shrimp Chowder (page 102)	Pear and Walnut Salad (page 115)
WEDNES-DAY	Tex-Mex Tofu Scramble	Turkey, Veggie, and Rice Soup (page 76)	Quick Red Beans and Rice (page 86)	Berries with Honeyed Green Tea Yogurt Sauce
THURSDAY	Tropical Smoothie (page 49)	White Bean and Bell Pepper Wraps (page 69)	Easy Corn and Shrimp Chowder	Pear and Walnut Salad
FRIDAY	Tropical Smoothie	Turkey, Veggie, and Rice Soup	Quick Red Beans and Rice	Homemade Apple-sauce (page 117) plus 2 tablespoons walnuts
SATURDAY	Orange Spice Whole-Grain French Toast (page 55)	White Bean and Bell Pepper Wraps	Hand-Cut Zoodles with Turkey Bolognese (page 95)	1 cup Rosemary Sweet Potato Chips (page 114)
SUNDAY	Egg and Spinach Scramble (page 59)	Turkey, Veggie, and Rice Soup	Turkey Burgers (page 90)	Homemade Applesauce plus 2 tablespoons walnuts

Shopping List

PRODUCE

- Apples (6)
- Arugula (1 bunch)
- Bell pepper, green (1)
- Bell peppers, red (4)
- Berries, mixed (2 pints)
- Celery stalks (4)
- Chives (1 bunch)
- Fennel bulb (1)
- Garlic (2 heads)
- Ginger (1 large piece)
- Lemons (3)
- Lettuce (1 head)
- Lime (1)
- Onion, red (1)
- Onions, yellow (4)
- Oranges (5)
- Pears (4)
- Pineapple (1)
- Rosemary (1 bunch)
- Spinach, baby, 1 (9-ounce) bag
- Sweet potatoes (2)
- Tarragon, fresh or dried
- Tomato, large (1)
- Zucchini, medium (8)

PROTEIN: MEAT, POULTRY, AND SEAFOOD

- Eggs (1 dozen)
- Salmon, 4 (4-ounce) fillets
- Shrimp, baby, cooked (12 ounces)
- Turkey breast, ground (3 pounds)

DAIRY

- ☐ Coconut milk, light, 1 (14-ounce) can
- ☐ Greek yogurt, dairy or nondairy, nonfat plain
- ☐ Milk, dairy or nondairy, low-fat plain

NUTS AND SEEDS

- ☐ Walnuts

CONDIMENTS, HERBS, SPICES, AND OILS

- ☐ Fish sauce
- ☐ Green tea powder
- ☐ Hot sauce, sugar-free
- ☐ Paprika, smoked
- ☐ Thyme, dried

BREADS AND GRAINS

- ☐ Bread, whole-grain (1 loaf)
- ☐ Hamburger buns, whole wheat (4)
- ☐ Rice, brown (cooked or uncooked)
- ☐ Tortillas, whole wheat (4)

CANNED, PACKAGED, AND PANTRY STAPLES

- ☐ Cannellini beans, 1 (15-ounce) can
- ☐ Corn, 1 (11-ounce) can
- ☐ Small red beans, 1 (15-ounce) can
- ☐ Tomatoes, crushed, 1 (28-ounce) can
- ☐ Vegetable broth, low-sodium (100 ounces)

SHOPPING TIPS

☐ Double-check the staples, produce, spices, and dairy lists before you shop, because you may have some left over from last week; replenish as needed.

☐ If you plan to make your own vegetable broth instead of buying it, you'll need to include broth ingredients on your shopping list and omit the canned broth.

☐ Some leftovers from last week will carry over to breakfast and lunch this week.

PREP AHEAD (SUNDAY)

☐ Make the broth if not using canned.

☐ Make the Honeyed Green Tea Yogurt Sauce and refrigerate for up to five days.

☐ Make the Turkey, Veggie, and Rice Soup and freeze in single servings.

PREP AHEAD (WEDNESDAY)

☐ Cook a large batch of rice for the Quick Red Beans and Rice and refrigerate it for up to five days or freeze for up to six months.

☐ Make the Homemade Applesauce and refrigerate it for up to five days or freeze for six months.

☐ Make the Rosemary Sweet Potato Chips and store them in an airtight container for up to one week.

Week 5

	BREAKFAST	LUNCH	DINNER	SNACK
MONDAY	Green Smoothie Bowl (page 50)	Lemon-Garlic Shrimp and Orzo Salad (page 80)	Black Bean Burritos (page 87) 2 tablespoons Guacamole (page 110)	*1 cup Rosemary Sweet Potato Chips* 1 ounce dark chocolate (optional treat)
TUESDAY	Apple-Cinnamon Overnight Oats (page 53)	Eggless Egg Salad Sandwiches (page 71)	Baked Chicken Tenders (page 89) *1 cup Rosemary Sweet Potato Chips*	1 orange plus ½ cup plain nonfat yogurt or nondairy yogurt
WEDNES-DAY	*Green Smoothie Bowl*	*Lemon-Garlic Shrimp and Orzo Salad*	Citrus-Soy Salmon and Veggie Packets (page 97) ¼ cup cooked brown rice	2 Cocoa and Cranberry Energy Balls (page 118)
THURSDAY	*Apple-Cinnamon Overnight Oats*	*Eggless Egg Salad Sandwiches*	Baked Cod with Lemon and Scallions (page 101) ½ baked sweet potato	Spicy Bean Dip (page 111) ¼ bell pepper, sliced
FRIDAY	Pumpkin Spice Smoothie (page 46)	Salmon Salad Lettuce Wraps (page 77)	Whole Wheat Pasta Puttanesca (page 88)	*1 cup Rosemary Sweet Potato Chips*
SATURDAY	Turkey Sausage and Sweet Potato Hash (page 61)	Soba Salad with Sesame Dressing (page 67)	Mustard Roasted Pork Tenderloin and Sweet Potatoes (page 96)	*2 Cocoa and Cranberry Energy Balls*
SUNDAY	Tex-Mex Tofu Scramble (page 60)	*Salmon Salad Lettuce Wraps*	Grilled Shrimp with Mango-Cucumber Salsa (page 104) ¼ cup cooked quinoa	*Spicy Bean Dip* ¼ bell pepper, sliced

Shopping List

PRODUCE

- ☐ Apple, green (1)
- ☐ Apples, dried
- ☐ Avocados (2)
- ☐ Banana (1)
- ☐ Basil (1 bunch)
- ☐ Bell pepper, red (1)
- ☐ Bell peppers, green (2)
- ☐ Berries, mixed (1 pint)
- ☐ Carrots (4)
- ☐ Cilantro (3 bunches)
- ☐ Cranberries, dried
- ☐ Cucumber (1 small)
- ☐ Fennel bulb (1)
- ☐ Garlic (2 heads)
- ☐ Jalapeños (3)
- ☐ Lemons (4)
- ☐ Lettuce, butter (1 head)
- ☐ Limes (12)
- ☐ Mango (1)
- ☐ Onions, red (3)
- ☐ Onions, yellow (2)
- ☐ Oranges (4)
- ☐ Parsley (1 bunch)
- ☐ Peas, fresh or frozen (1 pound)
- ☐ Scallions (2 bunches)
- ☐ Shallots (10)
- ☐ Spinach, baby, 1 (9-ounce) bag
- ☐ Sweet potatoes (7)
- ☐ Thyme (1 bunch)
- ☐ Tomatoes, cherry (1 pint)
- ☐ Tomatoes, large (6)
- ☐ Zucchini, medium (4)

PROTEIN: MEAT, POULTRY, AND SEAFOOD

- ☐ Chicken breast tenders (1 pound)
- ☐ Cod, skinless, 4 (4-ounce) fillets
- ☐ Pork tenderloin (1 pound)
- ☐ Salmon, Pacific, 4 (4-ounce) fillets
- ☐ Salmon, pink Pacific, 2 (3-ounce) cans or pouches

- ☐ Shrimp, baby, cooked (8 ounces)
- ☐ Shrimp, large (1 pound)
- ☐ Tofu, extra-firm (6 ounces)
- ☐ Tofu, silken, extra-firm (6 ounces)
- ☐ Turkey breast, ground (8 ounces)

DAIRY

- ☐ Milk, dairy or nondairy, low-fat plain
- ☐ Yogurt, dairy or nondairy, plain

NUTS AND SEEDS

- ☐ Almond butter
- ☐ Almonds, slivered
- ☐ Pepitas
- ☐ Sesame seeds

CONDIMENTS, HERBS, SPICES, AND OILS

- ☐ Almond flour
- ☐ Chinese hot mustard powder
- ☐ Chipotle chili powder
- ☐ Cocoa powder, unsweetened
- ☐ Mustard, Dijon
- ☐ Stevia

BREADS AND GRAINS

- ☐ Farfalle pasta, whole wheat, 1 (1-pound) box
- ☐ Oats, old-fashioned
- ☐ Orzo, whole wheat or gluten-free, 1 (16-ounce) box
- ☐ Quinoa
- ☐ Rice, brown
- ☐ Soba, 1 (9.5-ounce) package
- ☐ Tortillas, whole wheat

CANNED, PACKAGED, AND PANTRY STAPLES

☐ Black beans, 3 (15-ounce) cans

☐ Black olives, sliced,
2 (2.5-ounce) cans

☐ Capers

☐ Pinto beans, 1 (14-ounce) can

☐ Pumpkin puree, 1 (14-ounce) can

☐ Tomatoes, diced, 1 (15-ounce) can

TREATS

☐ Dark chocolate

☐ Red wine

SHOPPING TIPS

☐ Double-check the staples, produce, spices, and dairy lists before shopping because you may have some left over from last week; replenish as needed.

☐ If making your own vegetable broth, you'll need to include broth ingredients on your shopping list and omit the canned broth.

PREP AHEAD (SUNDAY)

☐ Cook the orzo for the Lemon-Garlic Shrimp and Orzo Salad and refrigerate it.

☐ Precook the quinoa and the brown rice, and refrigerate them for five days or freeze for up to six months.

PREP AHEAD (WEDNESDAY)

☐ Make the Cocoa and Cranberry Energy Balls and refrigerate them for up to five days or freeze them for up to six months.

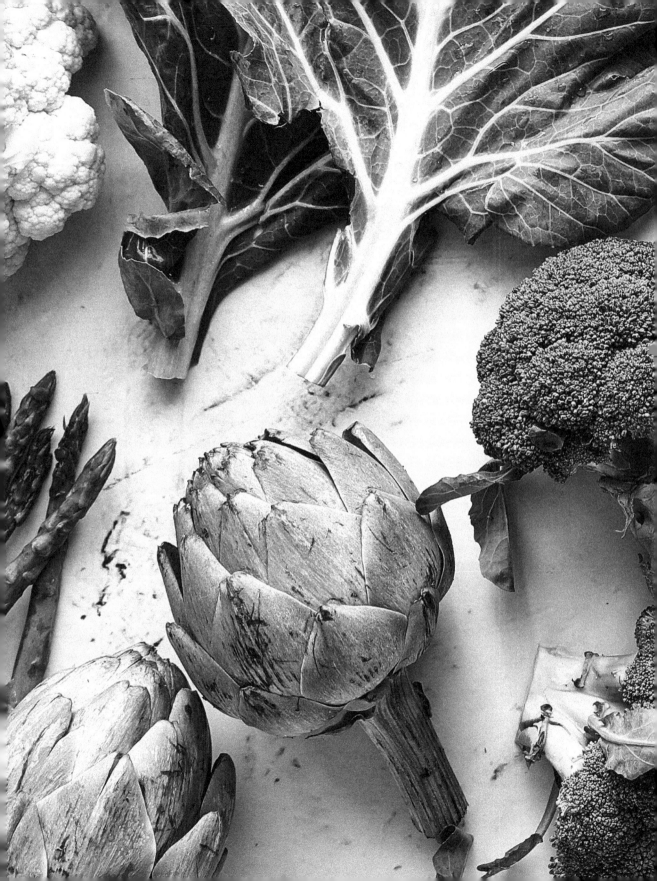

PART 02

75 METABOLISM-BOOSTING RECIPES

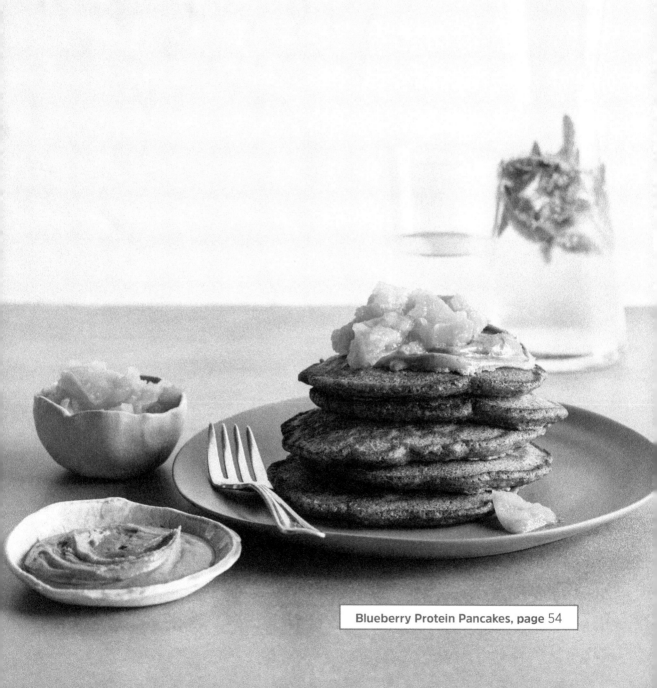

Blueberry Protein Pancakes, page 54

CHAPTER 3

BREAKFAST AND SMOOTHIES

Pumpkin Spice Smoothie

Grain-Free, Sugar-Free, Vegan

Serves 2 • **Prep time:** 5 minutes

You can easily make a larger batch of this lightly sweet smoothie to freeze for future breakfasts on the go. Pour the smoothie into ice cube trays and freeze. Divide the frozen cubes between two plastic zip-top bags and freeze for up to six months. To use, place the cubes in a blender with about ½ cup of water (or skim or nondairy milk) and blend until smooth.

1 cup unsweetened plain nondairy milk

1 packet stevia (¼ teaspoon or about 16 drops of liquid stevia)

2 cups canned pumpkin puree

¼ teaspoon vanilla extract

½ teaspoon Pumpkin Pie Spice Blend (page 131)

½ cup crushed ice

In a blender, combine the nondairy milk, stevia, pumpkin, vanilla, Pumpkin Pie Spice Blend, and ice and blend until smooth.

Tip: Boost the anti-inflammatory benefits of this smoothie by adding up to ½ teaspoon ground ginger or turmeric.

Per Serving: Calories: 123; Total fat: 2.5g; Saturated fat: 0g; Cholesterol: 0mg; Carbohydrates: 21g; Fiber: 6g; Protein: 3g

Gingerbread Smoothie

Grain-Free, Vegan

Serves 2 • **Prep time:** 10 minutes

This vegan smoothie has a surprising vegetable base–cauliflower rice. You can buy premade cauliflower rice in the produce, freezer, or rice section of your grocery store. Don't worry if you don't like cauliflower. It's disguised by the other ingredients to make a delicious, fruit-free smoothie.

1 herbal ginger tea bag

2 cups boiling water

2 cups cauliflower rice

½ teaspoon Pumpkin Pie Spice Blend (page 131)

1 tablespoon tahini

2 tablespoons black-strap molasses or pure maple syrup

½ teaspoon ground ginger

½ cup crushed ice

1. In a large measuring cup, steep the tea bag in the boiling water for 5 minutes. Discard the tea bag and let the tea cool.

2. In a blender, combine the cooled ginger tea, cauliflower rice, Pumpkin Pie Spice Blend, tahini, molasses, ginger, and ice and blend until smooth.

Tip: Adjust the sweetness level by using more or less molasses. You can also make this entirely sugar-free by replacing the molasses or syrup with 1 to 2 packets of stevia (¼ teaspoon or about 16 drops of liquid stevia = 1 packet).

Per Serving: Calories: 138; Total fat: 4g; Saturated fat: 0.5g; Cholesterol: 0mg; Carbohydrates: 19g; Fiber: 2.5g; Protein: 4g

Cocoa Chia Smoothie

Grain-Free, Sugar-Free, Vegan

Serves 2 • **Prep time:** 20 minutes

Make sure you choose unsweetened cocoa powder for this smoothie. While this is a fruit-free smoothie, you can also add half a banana for some sweetness and additional flavor. Don't skip the step of soaking the chia in the milk, as this thickens the smoothie.

2 cups unsweetened plain nondairy milk

¼ cup chia seeds

2 tablespoons unsweetened cocoa powder

¼ teaspoon vanilla extract

2 packets stevia (½ teaspoon or about 32 drops of liquid stevia)

1 cup crushed ice

1. In a blender, combine the nondairy milk and chia seeds and let the mixture rest for 15 minutes.

2. Add the cocoa powder, vanilla, stevia, and ice and blend until smooth.

Tip: Want this thicker? Add half an avocado before blending.

Per Serving: Calories: 153; Total fat: 10g; Saturated fat: 1g; Cholesterol: 0mg; Carbohydrates: 13g; Fiber: 9g; Protein: 6g

Tropical Smoothie

Grain-Free, Sugar-Free, Vegan

Serves 2 • **Prep time:** 5 minutes

If you want a fruity smoothie that's naturally sweet without any added sweeteners or sugar, then this tropical delight will transport you to the islands. Made with fresh pineapple and coconut milk, it has the classic flavors of a piña colada minus the rum. It's fast, easy, and delicious.

2 cups fresh pineapple chunks

1 cup canned light coconut milk

1 cup unsweetened plain nondairy milk

2 tablespoons tahini

½ cup crushed ice

In a blender, combine the pineapple, coconut milk, nondairy milk, tahini, and ice and blend until smooth.

Tip: Save time by purchasing chopped pineapple from the salad bar at the grocery store or frozen (unsweetened) chopped pineapple. If you use frozen pineapple, reduce the ice to ¼ cup.

Per Serving: Calories: 184; Total fat: 15g; Saturated fat: 5.5g; Cholesterol: 0mg; Carbohydrates: 10g; Fiber: 1.5g; Protein: 3g

Green Smoothie Bowl

Grain-Free, Vegan

Serves 2 • **Prep time:** 15 minutes

Smoothie bowls make beautiful, Instagram-worthy breakfasts, and this colorful version is no exception. The deep green of the smoothie contrasts nicely with the mixed berries as garnish. It's lightly sweet, highly satisfying, and deeply nourishing. In short, it's a great way to start your day.

2½ cups packed baby spinach

1 green apple, cored and chopped

1 small banana, peeled

½ avocado, pitted and peeled

½ cup unsweetened plain nondairy milk

1 tablespoon pure maple syrup

½ cup mixed berries

¼ cup toasted slivered almonds (optional)

1 teaspoon sesame seeds

1. In a blender, combine the spinach, apple, banana, avocado, nondairy milk, and maple syrup and blend until smooth.

2. Pour the mixture equally into two bowls. Garnish with the berries, almonds (if using), and sesame seeds.

Per Serving: Calories: 226; Total fat: 7g; Saturated fat: 1g; Cholesterol: 0mg; Carbohydrates: 40g; Fiber: 9g; Protein: 4g

Golden Milk Chia Breakfast Pudding with Blueberries

Grain-Free, Vegan

Serves 2 • **Prep time:** 15 minutes, plus overnight to set • **Cook time:** 5 minutes

Something magical happens when you soak chia seeds in liquid: They expand and thicken and create a pudding with a tapioca-like consistency. Chia is a nutritious food, with healthy anti-inflammatory omega-3 fatty acids that work synergistically with the anti-inflammatory golden milk. Make this the night before, refrigerate, and the next morning you'll have a tasty breakfast that's ready to go.

1 cup unsweetened plain nondairy milk

¼ teaspoon ground turmeric

¼ teaspoon ground ginger

2 tablespoons pure maple syrup

4 tablespoons chia seeds

½ cup fresh blueberries

1. In a saucepan, combine the nondairy milk, turmeric, ginger, and maple syrup and bring to a simmer, stirring constantly, over medium heat.

2. Divide the chia seeds between two glass jars or bowls. Remove the saucepan from the heat, pour the mixture into the two glass jars or bowls, and stir until combined. Refrigerate overnight.

3. Serve garnished with the blueberries.

Per Serving: Calories: 195; Total fat: 8g; Saturated fat: 0.5g; Cholesterol: 0mg; Carbohydrates: 28g; Fiber: 8g; Protein: 4g

Cranberry-Ginger Oatmeal

Vegan

Serves 2 • **Prep time:** 15 minutes • **Cook time:** 5 minutes

Cranberries are a great source of antioxidants and fiber, so they're anti-inflammatory, nutritious, and filling. Likewise, ginger is an anti-inflammatory food that also works as a mild appetite suppressant and digestive stimulant. That makes this simple breakfast a morning superfood when you're trying to kick-start your metabolism.

2 cups unsweetened plain nondairy milk

1 teaspoon ground ginger

1 tablespoon pure maple syrup

Pinch sea salt

1 cup old-fashioned oats

½ cup dried cranberries

¼ cup pepitas (hulled pumpkin seeds)

1. In a small saucepan, combine the nondairy milk, ginger, maple syrup, and salt and bring to a boil over medium-high heat.

2. Add the oats and cook, stirring occasionally, for 5 minutes.

3. Spoon the mixture into two bowls. Garnish with the dried cranberries and pepitas and serve.

Tip: Add orange flavor by replacing ½ cup of the milk with freshly squeezed orange juice. Garnish with a light grating of orange zest.

Per Serving: Calories: 390; Total fat: 14g; Saturated fat: 2g; Cholesterol: 0mg; Carbohydrates: 60g; Fiber: 6.5g; Protein: 11g

Apple-Cinnamon Overnight Oats

Vegan

Serves 2 • **Prep time:** 15 minutes, plus overnight to set

This is another recipe that allows you to prepare your breakfast the night before so it's ready to go when you get out of bed in the morning. You can use any single-serving bowls, although mason jars make a portable and cute presentation. Keep it refrigerated and give it a good stir before serving to make sure all the ingredients are well mixed.

1 cup old-fashioned oats

2 tablespoons chia seeds

½ teaspoon ground cinnamon

½ cup chopped dried apples

2 tablespoons pure maple syrup

1 cup unsweetened plain nondairy milk

2 tablespoons pepitas (hulled pumpkin seeds)

1. In a small bowl, combine the oats, chia seeds, cinnamon, and apples and mix well.

2. Divide the mixture between two single-serving containers, such as bowls or jars.

3. In a glass measuring cup, whisk together the maple syrup and nondairy milk. Pour ½ cup into each of the bowls and stir well.

4. Cover and refrigerate overnight.

5. Remove from the refrigerator and stir. Garnish with the pepitas and serve.

Tip: You can boost the apple flavor by replacing ½ cup of the milk with ½ cup of unfiltered apple juice.

Per Serving: Calories: 323; Total fat: 11g; Saturated fat: 1.5g; Cholesterol: 0mg; Carbohydrates: 47g; Fiber: 10g; Protein: 11g

Blueberry Protein Pancakes

Grain-Free, Sugar-Free

Makes 8 pancakes • **Prep time:** 15 minutes • **Cook time:** 15 minutes

These pancakes make a great grain-free option for when you want a stick-with-you breakfast. Top them with pure maple syrup or your favorite nut butter, eat them plain, or have them with Homemade Applesauce (page 117). It's a delicious and filling way to start your day with a nutritious breakfast.

½ cup sugar-free vegan vanilla protein powder

¼ cup almond flour

1 teaspoon baking powder

¼ cup unsweetened plain nondairy milk

1 egg

¼ cup fresh or frozen blueberries

½ tablespoon avocado oil

1. In a small bowl, whisk together the protein powder, almond flour, and baking powder.

2. In another small bowl or glass measuring cup, whisk together the nondairy milk and egg.

3. Add the wet ingredients to the dry ingredients and fold with a rubber spatula until just combined.

4. Fold in the blueberries.

5. In a nonstick skillet, heat the oil over medium-high heat.

6. Spoon 2 tablespoons of the batter into the skillet for each pancake. You will need to make them in batches. Cook until bubbles form on top of the pancake, about 3 minutes. Flip with a spatula and cook on the other side until browned, about 3 minutes more.

Tip: Use an unsweetened flavored protein powder such as coffee or cocoa for an interesting and flavorful twist.

Per Serving (2 pancakes): Calories: 126; Total fat: 7g; Saturated fat: 1g; Cholesterol: 46mg; Carbohydrates: 4g; Fiber: 1.5g; Protein: 13g

Orange Spice Whole-Grain French Toast

Sugar-Free

Serves 4 • **Prep time:** 15 minutes • **Cook time:** 15 minutes

If you prefer French toast to pancakes, this is an easy and delicious choice. It's scrumptious without any toppings, but you can spoon Homemade Applesauce (page 117), sliced fruit, honey, nut or seed butter, or pure maple syrup over the top.

4 eggs, beaten

1 cup unsweetened plain nondairy milk

Grated zest and juice of ½ orange

½ teaspoon vanilla

½ teaspoon ground cinnamon

4 slices whole-grain bread or whole-grain gluten-free bread

½ teaspoon avocado oil

1. In a medium bowl, whisk together the eggs, non-dairy milk, orange zest, orange juice, vanilla, and cinnamon.

2. In a shallow baking dish, arrange the bread in a single layer and pour the egg mixture over the top. Allow it to soak for about 5 minutes.

3. In a nonstick skillet, heat the oil over medium-high heat, swirling the pan to coat it with the oil.

4. Remove the bread from the baking dish and place it in the skillet. Cook until well browned, about 5 minutes per side.

Tip: Use a rasp-style grater to zest the orange. Take care to only grate the orange part of the orange peel. The white part just below the orange part of the peel, called the pith, is bitter.

Per Serving: Calories: 181; Total fat: 6.5g; Saturated fat: 1.5g; Cholesterol: 167mg; Carbohydrates: 21g; Fiber: 2g; Protein: 11g

Spicy Avocado and Pepita Toast

Sugar-Free, Vegan

Serves 2 • **Prep time:** 5 minutes • **Cook time:** 5 minutes

There's a reason avocado toast has become such a popular dish—it's nutritious and filling, and mashed avocado makes a great, creamy, more nutritious replacement for butter or margarine. For best results, mash the avocado just before you make the toast; otherwise, the avocado may brown from oxidation. If you do premake the avocado, put it in a dish with plastic wrap touching the surface to keep any air out.

½ avocado, pitted, peeled, and chopped

1 teaspoon freshly squeezed lemon juice

¼ teaspoon sea salt

½ garlic clove, minced

⅛ to ¼ teaspoon cayenne pepper

2 slices of whole-grain bread or whole-grain gluten-free bread, toasted

4 cherry tomatoes, halved

2 tablespoons pepitas (hulled pumpkin seeds)

1. In a medium bowl, combine the avocado, lemon juice, salt, garlic, and ⅛ teaspoon of cayenne (plus more if you like it spicy) and mash with a fork.

2. Spread the mixture on the toasted bread.

3. Garnish with the tomatoes and pepitas and serve.

Tip: Always start with the smallest amount of cayenne first. Taste and adjust as needed, adding a little bit at a time to achieve the right amount of seasoning. You can also substitute chipotle chili powder for a smokier flavor.

Per Serving: Calories: 258; Total fat: 15g; Saturated fat: 2g; Cholesterol: 0mg; Carbohydrates: 25g; Fiber: 7.5g; Protein: 10g

Broccoli and Bell Pepper Frittata Muffins

Grain-Free, Sugar-Free

Makes 12 muffins • **Prep time:** 10 minutes • **Cook time:** 20 minutes

These colorful, antioxidant-rich muffins are easy to make ahead, so you'll always have a tasty breakfast ready to go. You can freeze them in single servings (2 muffins) in a zip-top plastic bag for up to six months. Thaw and reheat in the oven at 350°F for about 20 minutes or in the microwave for about 1 minute.

1 tablespoon avocado oil, plus additional for oiling the muffin tins

1 shallot, peeled and minced

2 cups chopped broccoli florets and stems

1 red bell pepper, stemmed, seeded, and chopped

12 large eggs, beaten

2 tablespoons unsweetened plain nondairy milk

½ teaspoon garlic powder

1 teaspoon Dijon mustard

½ teaspoon sea salt

¼ teaspoon freshly ground black pepper

1. Preheat the oven to 350°F. Brush a 12-cup nonstick muffin tin with avocado oil.

2. In a large nonstick skillet, heat the oil over medium-high heat until it shimmers. Add the shallot, broccoli, and bell pepper and cook, stirring occasionally, until softened, 5 to 7 minutes. Let cool and divide equally between the muffin cups.

3. In a large bowl, whisk together the eggs, non-dairy milk, garlic powder, mustard, salt, and black pepper. Ladle or pour the mixture over the vegetables in the muffin cups.

4. Bake for 15 to 20 minutes, or until set.

Tip: You can omit the oil in the muffin tins by lining them with silicone muffin liners, which are available online, at grocery stores in the baking aisle, or from kitchen stores.

Per Serving (2 muffins): Calories: 207; Total fat: 14g; Saturated fat: 3.5g; Cholesterol: 372mg; Carbohydrates: 5g; Fiber: 1.5g; Protein: 14g

Breakfast Burritos

Sugar-Free

Serves 2 • **Prep time:** 15 minutes • **Cook time:** 20 minutes

These burritos are fast and easy to make. For a spicier version, you can add a seeded and chopped jalapeño when you cook the onion, and you can also add a pinch of cayenne or chipotle chili powder to the egg mixture—up to ¼ teaspoon depending on how much heat you want.

2 (8-inch) whole-grain tortillas

4 eggs, beaten

¼ teaspoon ground cumin

¼ teaspoon garlic powder

¼ teaspoon chili powder

¼ teaspoon sea salt

1 teaspoon avocado oil

¼ red onion, minced

1 cup Pico de Gallo (page 124)

¼ cup Buttermilk Ranch Dressing (page 125)

1. Preheat the oven to 350°F. Wrap the tortillas in aluminum foil and warm them in the oven for 15 minutes.

2. In a medium bowl, whisk together the eggs, cumin, garlic powder, chili powder, and salt. Set aside.

3. In a medium nonstick skillet, heat the oil over medium-high heat until it shimmers. Add the onion and cook, stirring occasionally, until soft, 3 to 5 minutes.

4. Add the egg mixture and cook, scrambling with a spoon, until the eggs are set, 3 to 5 minutes.

5. Spoon the egg mixture equally into the tortillas. Top each with half of the Pico de Gallo and 2 tablespoons of the Buttermilk Ranch Dressing.

6. Fold in the sides, roll up the tortillas around the filling, and serve.

Tip: Add a few slices of avocado to each burrito and up to 2 tablespoons of chopped fresh cilantro to boost the flavors if you wish.

Per Serving: Calories: 293; Total fat: 15g; Saturated fat: 3.5g; Cholesterol: 372mg; Carbohydrates: 29g; Fiber: 14g; Protein: 22g

Egg and Spinach Scramble

Grain-Free, Sugar-Free

Serves 2 ● **Prep time:** 10 minutes ● **Cook time:** 10 minutes

Eggs reheat well in the microwave, so you can make this ahead of time and refrigerate it for up to three days. To reheat, cover and microwave it on high for 1 minute. Feel free to substitute other dark, leafy greens for the spinach—try an equal amount of kale, Swiss chard, or another green.

1 tablespoon avocado oil

3 scallions, white and green parts, minced

2 cups baby spinach leaves

4 eggs, beaten

½ teaspoon sea salt

¼ teaspoon freshly ground black pepper

½ teaspoon Dijon mustard

1. In a large nonstick skillet, heat the oil over medium-high heat until it shimmers.

2. Add the scallions and cook, stirring occasionally, until soft, about 2 minutes.

3. Add the spinach and cook, stirring occasionally, until soft, 2 to 3 minutes.

4. In a small bowl, whisk together the eggs, salt, black pepper, and mustard.

5. Add the mixture to the skillet and cook, scrambling with a spatula, until the eggs are firm, about 3 minutes. Serve immediately.

Tip: Add ¼ teaspoon of ground cumin and ¼ teaspoon of chili powder to the eggs and omit the mustard for a slightly spicier, Tex-Mex-inspired version.

Per Serving: Calories: 224; Total fat: 16g; Saturated fat: 4g; Cholesterol: 372mg; Carbohydrates: 4g; Fiber: 1.5g; Protein: 14g

Tex-Mex Tofu Scramble

Grain-Free, Sugar-Free, Vegan

Serves 2 • **Prep time:** 15 minutes • **Cook time:** 20 minutes

Tofu makes a great vegan substitute for eggs in a morning breakfast scramble. Use extra-firm silken tofu for best results. You can make this ahead and reheat it in the microwave. It will keep, tightly sealed, in the refrigerator for about five days. Reheat in the microwave for 1 minute.

1 tablespoon avocado oil

6 ounces extra-firm silken tofu, chopped (see Tip)

Pico de Gallo (page 124)

½ cup canned black beans, drained

Juice of 1 lime

1 teaspoon chili powder

¼ teaspoon ground cumin

½ teaspoon sea salt

1. In a large nonstick skillet, heat the oil over medium-high heat.

2. Add the tofu and cook, stirring occasionally, until it starts to turn golden, 3 to 5 minutes.

3. Add the Pico de Gallo and beans and cook, stirring occasionally, for 5 minutes.

4. In a small bowl, whisk together the lime juice, chili powder, cumin, and salt, then add the mixture to the skillet. Cook, stirring, for 2 minutes more. Serve hot.

Tip: You can make the tofu even firmer by removing excess moisture. To do this, place the block of tofu in a colander in the sink and put a plate on top, pressing directly down on the tofu. Use a can to weigh the plate down and let it sit in the sink for 30 minutes to drain any excess water. This step isn't necessary, but it creates a better texture for the end product.

Per Serving: Calories: 221; Total fat: 10g; Saturated fat: 1g; Cholesterol: 0mg; Carbohydrates: 24g; Fiber: 7g; Protein: 12g

Turkey Sausage and Sweet Potato Hash

Grain-Free, Sugar-Free

Serves 6 • **Prep time:** 15 minutes • **Cook time:** 30 minutes

You can enjoy Sunday brunch and still boost your metabolism with this delicious hash. It's easy to make your own sage turkey breakfast sausage, and sweet potatoes add color and plenty of vitamin A. This serves 6, but leftovers reheat well for fast weekday meals. Store it in your refrigerator in an airtight container for up to five days.

8 ounces ground turkey breast

1 teaspoon ground sage

1 teaspoon sea salt, divided

¼ teaspoon freshly ground black pepper, divided

¼ teaspoon red chili flakes

2 tablespoons avocado oil

2 sweet potatoes, peeled and cut into ¼-inch cubes

1 red onion, chopped

1 green bell pepper, stemmed, seeded, and chopped

1 garlic clove, minced

1. Preheat the oven to 400°F. Line a rimmed baking sheet with aluminum foil.

2. In a medium bowl, combine the ground turkey, sage, ½ teaspoon of salt, ⅛ teaspoon of black pepper, and the red chili flakes and mix well.

3. Form the mixture into 8 patties and place them on the prepared baking sheet. Bake until cooked through (an internal temperature of 185°F), about 30 minutes.

4. While the sausage cooks, in a large nonstick skillet, heat the oil over medium-high heat until it shimmers.

5. Add the potatoes, onion, bell pepper, remaining ½ teaspoon of salt, and remaining ⅛ teaspoon of black pepper, cover, and cook, stirring occasionally, until the potatoes are soft and beginning to brown, 15 to 20 minutes.

6. Remove the sausage from the oven and cut it into bite-size pieces. Add it to the skillet with the potatoes. Add the garlic and cook, stirring, for 1 minute more.

Per Serving: Calories: 135; Total fat: 5.5g; Saturated fat: 0.5g; Cholesterol: 24mg; Carbohydrates: 12g; Fiber: 2g; Protein: 10g

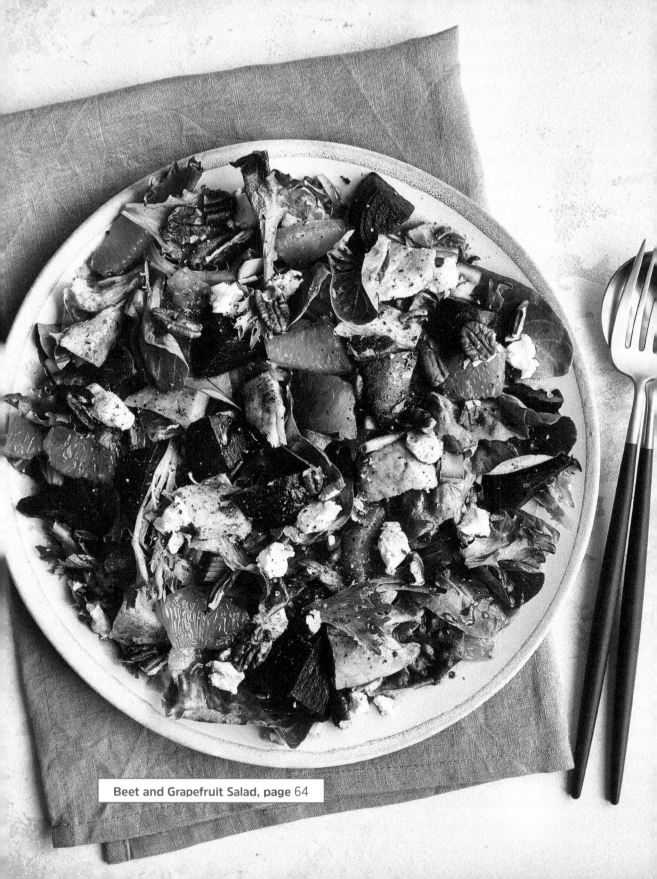

Beet and Grapefruit Salad, page 64

LUNCH

Beet and Grapefruit Salad

Grain-Free, Sugar-Free

Serves 2 • **Prep time:** 20 minutes • **Cook time:** 20 minutes

Grapefruit contains naringenin. What's that? It's an antioxidant your body uses to help process insulin, and better insulin use promotes a faster metabolism. Eating grapefruit also lowers your insulin levels, so it's a great metabolism-boosting ingredient to add to a number of dishes.

2 beets, greens removed, peeled and cut into ¼-inch slices

3 tablespoons avocado oil, divided

¾ teaspoon sea salt, divided

2 cups chopped cooked boneless, skinless chicken breast

2 cups mixed greens

1 grapefruit, peeled and chopped

¼ red onion, diced

½ cup crushed pecans

¼ cup balsamic vinegar

½ teaspoon Dijon mustard

1. Preheat the oven to 425°F.

2. Place the beet slices on a rimmed baking sheet in a single layer and brush them with 1 tablespoon of oil. Sprinkle the beets with ½ teaspoon of salt. Roast until soft, about 20 minutes. Let cool. Cut the slices into quarters and transfer them to a large bowl.

3. Add the cooked chicken breast, greens, grape-fruit, onion, and pecans to the bowl and toss until mixed.

4. In a small bowl, whisk together the 2 remaining tablespoons of oil, the remaining ¼ teaspoon of salt, the vinegar, and the mustard. Pour the dressing over the salad and toss it just before serving.

Tip: Add 2 tablespoons of crumbled low-fat feta cheese for saltiness and tang.

Per Serving: Calories: 633; Total fat: 44g; Saturated fat: 5g; Cholesterol: 85mg; Carbohydrates: 31g; Fiber: 7.5g; Protein: 32g

Fiesta Quinoa and Bell Pepper Salad

Sugar-Free, Vegan

Serves 4 • **Prep time:** 10 minutes • **Cook time:** 20 minutes

This colorful salad combines the toothsome texture of quinoa with the crunch of fresh bell peppers and the tang of a flavorful vinaigrette for a true taste explosion. You can combine the entire salad ahead of time and store it in the refrigerator for up to five days. Feel free to add 2 ounces of protein per serving, such as chopped tofu, tempeh, or baby shrimp.

2 cups Vegetable Broth (page 130)

1 cup quinoa, rinsed

¾ teaspoon sea salt, divided

1 red bell pepper, stemmed, seeded, and chopped

1 yellow bell pepper, stemmed, seeded, and chopped

4 scallions, white and green parts, cut into slices

¼ cup apple cider vinegar

2 tablespoons avocado oil

1 garlic clove, minced

1 teaspoon Dijon mustard

1. In a medium saucepan, combine the Vegetable Broth, quinoa, and ½ teaspoon of salt and bring to a boil over medium-high heat.

2. Lower the heat to medium-low and simmer, stirring occasionally, until the liquid is absorbed, 10 to 15 minutes. Fluff the quinoa with a fork and let it cool.

3. In a large bowl, combine the cooked quinoa, red and yellow bell peppers, and scallions and toss until mixed.

4. In a small bowl, whisk together the vinegar, oil, remaining ¼ teaspoon of salt, garlic, and mustard. Pour over the quinoa and toss until combined.

Tip: Always rinse quinoa before cooking. Place it in a fine-mesh sieve in the sink and run water through it, rubbing the grains between your fingers. This removes saponins on the grain's surface, which impart bitter flavors.

Per Serving: Calories: 249; Total fat: 10g; Saturated fat: 1g; Cholesterol: 0mg; Carbohydrates: 34g; Fiber: 4.5g; Protein: 7g

Whole Wheat Pasta Salad

Sugar-Free, Vegan

Serves 4 • **Prep time:** 20 minutes • **Cook time:** 10 minutes

Bowtie pasta shapes are fun for this salad, but you can also use rotini whole-grain pasta or even macaroni elbows. You can make it gluten-free by substituting your favorite gluten-free pasta. It will keep in the refrigerator in an airtight container for up to five days, so it's perfect to make ahead.

1 (8-ounce) box whole-wheat bowtie pasta

¼ red onion, finely chopped

½ cup sliced black olives, drained and rinsed

1 red bell pepper, stemmed, seeded, and finely chopped

10 fresh basil leaves, torn into pieces

¼ cup avocado oil

¾ cup apple cider vinegar

½ teaspoon sea salt

½ teaspoon Dijon mustard

2 garlic cloves, minced

1. Fill a large pot with water and bring it to a boil over high heat. Add the pasta and cook according to the package instructions. Drain the pasta and let it cool.

2. In a large bowl, mix the cooked pasta, onion, olives, bell pepper, and basil leaves.

3. In a medium bowl, whisk together the oil, vinegar, salt, mustard, and garlic. Pour the mixture over the pasta salad and toss until mixed.

Tip: Add 8 ounces of cooked lean protein, such as shrimp, salmon, or tofu, to the salad to make it a hearty dinner.

Per Serving: Calories: 394; Total fat: 19g; Saturated fat: 2g; Cholesterol: 0mg; Carbohydrates: 50g; Fiber: 7g; Protein: 10g

Soba Salad with Sesame Dressing

Grain-Free, Sugar-Free, Vegan

Serves 4 • **Prep time:** 15 minutes • **Cook time:** 10 minutes

Soba are Japanese noodles made from buckwheat or a combination of buckwheat and whole wheat. In spite of its name, buckwheat is not a grain, so soba are gluten-free (as long as they're made only with buckwheat). They're loaded with fiber, which makes them stick with you longer than other foods. This can help you manage your appetite.

1 (9½-ounce) package soba

2 carrots, peeled and grated

1 cup fresh peas (or frozen and thawed)

8 scallions, white and green parts, thinly sliced

2 tablespoons tahini

1 garlic clove, minced

¼ teaspoon sesame oil

½ teaspoon Chinese hot mustard powder

Juice of 3 limes

½ teaspoon sea salt

1. Bring a large pot of water to a boil over high heat. Add the soba and cook according to the package instructions. Drain the noodles and let them cool.

2. In a large bowl, toss together the cooked soba, carrots, peas, and scallions.

3. In a small bowl or glass measuring cup, whisk together the tahini, garlic, sesame oil, mustard powder, lime juice, and salt. Add the dressing to the salad and toss until combined.

Tip: Boost the sesame flavor by garnishing this salad with 2 tablespoons of sesame seeds. For more crunch, you can also garnish the salad with 2 tablespoons of chopped cashews, peanuts, or almonds.

Per Serving: Calories: 350; Total fat: 5g; Saturated fat: 0.5g; Cholesterol: 0mg; Carbohydrates: 67g; Fiber: 6.5g; Protein: 17g

Veggie and Hummus Pitas

Sugar-Free, Vegan

Serves 2 • **Prep time:** 10 minutes

Here is a vegan sandwich that will make a flavorful lunch or snack. Feel free to stuff in as many leafy greens or other vegetables as you wish, or follow the recipe exactly as written. The result is a crunchy, creamy sandwich, rich with the fragrance of lemon, sesame, and garlic.

1 (8-inch) whole wheat pita, halved

4 tablespoons Hummus (page 108)

½ red bell pepper, stemmed, seeded, and thinly sliced

¼ red onion, thinly sliced

½ cup chopped kale

4 cherry tomatoes, halved

2 tablespoons pepitas (hulled pumpkin seeds)

1. Spread the inside of each pita half with 2 tablespoons of the Hummus.

2. In a bowl, toss together the bell pepper, onion, kale, tomatoes, and pepitas.

3. Divide the mixture equally between the two pita pockets.

Per Serving (1 pita half): Calories: 236; Total fat: 9.5g; Saturated fat: 1.5g; Cholesterol: 0mg; Carbohydrates: 31g; Fiber: 6g; Protein: 9g

White Bean and Bell Pepper Wraps

Sugar-Free, Vegan

Serves 4 • **Prep time:** 15 minutes

This simple wrap has an explosion of flavors and textures thanks to the peppery bite of the arugula, the sweet flavor of the bell peppers, and the creamy notes of the white bean puree. You can make the puree in a blender or use a food processor. You may wish to add a little water to make it a more spreadable consistency.

1 (15-ounce) can cannellini beans, drained and rinsed

1 tablespoon avocado oil

Grated zest of ½ orange

Juice of 1 orange

2 tablespoons chopped fresh tarragon

½ teaspoon sea salt

Pinch red chili flakes

4 (8-inch) whole wheat tortillas

2 red bell peppers, stemmed, seeded, and cut into slices

1 cup arugula

1. In a blender, combine the beans, oil, orange zest, orange juice, tarragon, salt, and red chili flakes. Blend until smooth, adding a little water if needed to achieve the desired consistency.

2. Spread the mixture onto the tortillas and top it with the bell peppers and arugula. Wrap up the tortillas and serve.

Tip: If you can't find fresh tarragon, you can substitute 1 teaspoon of dried tarragon in the puree.

Per Serving: Calories: 217; Total fat: 6.5g; Saturated fat: 0.5g; Cholesterol: 0mg; Carbohydrates: 38g; Fiber: 20g; Protein: 14g

Tofu and Veggie Stir-Fry Wraps

Sugar-Free, Vegan

Serves 2 • **Prep time:** 15 minutes, plus 1 hour to marinate
Cook time: 10 minutes

You can enjoy these wraps with warmed ingredients or, if you're eating on the fly, they're good cold as well. If you're packing these in your lunch, you may want to pack the tortillas separately from the stir-fry. Then you can either add it cold to the wrap or warm it in the microwave before wrapping.

6 ounces extra-firm silken tofu, cut into ½-inch pieces

Citrus-Soy Marinade (page 129), divided

1 tablespoon avocado oil

6 scallions, white and green parts, chopped

1 teaspoon grated fresh ginger

2 cups chopped kale

2 garlic cloves, minced

¼ teaspoon sesame oil

2 (8-inch) whole wheat tortillas

¼ cup bean sprouts

1. In a zip-top plastic bag, combine the tofu with all but 2 tablespoons of the Citrus-Soy Marinade. Seal the bag and refrigerate for at least 1 hour and up to 4 hours.

2. Remove the tofu from the marinade and pat it dry with paper towels.

3. In a large nonstick skillet, heat the avocado oil over medium-high heat until it shimmers. Add the tofu, scallions, ginger, and kale and cook, stirring occasionally, until the tofu is browned and the vegetables are softened, about 5 minutes.

4. Add the garlic and sesame oil and cook, stirring constantly, for 30 seconds. Add the remaining 2 tablespoons of Citrus-Soy Marinade and cook, stirring, for 2 minutes more.

5. Let cool or keep warm and spoon the mixture into the tortillas. Top with the bean sprouts, wrap up the tortillas, and serve.

Tip: To give the wraps even more fresh flavor, add up to 2 tablespoons of chopped fresh cilantro per wrap when you add the bean sprouts. For a spicier wrap, you can also replace the sesame oil with an equal amount of sesame-chili oil.

Per Serving: Calories: 278; Total fat: 17g; Saturated fat: 1.5g; Cholesterol: 0mg; Carbohydrates: 28g; Fiber: 14g; Protein: 18g

Eggless Egg Salad Sandwiches

Sugar-Free, Vegan

Serves 2 • **Prep time:** 15 minutes

You won't miss the eggs in this vegan version of an egg salad sandwich. It's easy to make gluten-free by using gluten-free bread, and it's a great on-the-go meal. If you make it ahead and take it for lunch, don't put the egg salad on the bread until you're ready to eat. That way the bread won't get soggy.

6 ounces extra-firm tofu, drained, patted dry, and cut into ¼-inch cubes

2 scallions, white and green parts, finely chopped

¼ cup unsweetened plain nondairy yogurt

1 tablespoon Dijon mustard

¼ teaspoon ground turmeric

½ teaspoon sea salt

⅛ teaspoon freshly ground black pepper

4 slices whole wheat or gluten-free bread

1. In a large bowl, combine the tofu and scallions.

2. In a smaller bowl, whisk together the yogurt, mustard, turmeric, salt, and black pepper.

3. Add the yogurt mixture to the tofu mixture and mix well.

4. Spoon half of the mixture onto each of 2 slices of bread. Top with the remaining 2 slices. Cut the sandwiches in half and serve.

Tip: Peas add color, texture, and earthy flavor to this sandwich, so feel free to stir up to ½ cup of shelled fresh peas into the tofu mixture.

Per Serving: Calories: 356; Total fat: 8.5g; Saturated fat: 1.5g; Cholesterol: 0mg; Carbohydrates: 48g; Fiber: 6g; Protein: 17g

Spicy Broccoli and Chicken Slaw

Grain-Free, Sugar-Free

Serves 4 • **Prep time:** 10 minutes, plus 3 hours to marinate
Cook time: 25 minutes

Using premade broccoli slaw (you can find bags of it with the bagged salad at the grocery store) saves lots of time when you want to make this crunchy and satisfying salad. To make it ahead, roast the chicken, let it cool, and cut it into pieces. Whisk up the dressing and then toss all the components together just before serving.

Citrus-Soy Marinade (page 129)

2 (8-ounce) boneless, skinless chicken breasts

1 (9-ounce) bag broccoli slaw

4 scallions, white and green parts, cut into slices

Cilantro-Lime Dressing (page 126)

¼ teaspoon Chinese hot mustard powder

¼ teaspoon sugar-free hot sauce (optional)

1 tablespoon sesame seeds

1. In a zip-top plastic bag, combine the Citrus-Soy Marinade and the chicken breasts. Seal the bag and refrigerate for 3 hours.

2. Preheat the oven to 425°F.

3. Remove the chicken from the marinade and pat it dry with a paper towel. Place the chicken in a baking dish and roast for 20 to 30 minutes, or until the chicken reaches an internal temperature of 165°F. Remove the chicken from the oven and let it cool. Cut it into slices.

4. In a large bowl, combine the broccoli slaw, chicken, and scallions and toss until combined.

5. In a small bowl, whisk together the Cilantro-Lime Dressing, mustard powder, and hot sauce (if using). Pour over the slaw and toss until combined.

6. Sprinkle the sesame seeds over the top and serve.

Tip: You can make this a more traditional slaw by using shredded cabbage in place of the broccoli slaw.

Per Serving: Calories: 309; Total fat: 19g; Saturated fat: 2.5g; Cholesterol: 63mg; Carbohydrates: 8g; Fiber: 2.5g; Protein: 25g

Chicken and Black Bean Salad Lettuce Cups

Grain-Free, Sugar-Free

Serves 4 • **Prep time:** 10 minutes, plus 3 hours to marinate
Cook time: 20 minutes

The protein found in chicken and beans can help keep you energized and filled up for hours, and the black beans in this recipe also contain plenty of fiber for satiation. Legumes such as black beans contain arginine, which is an amino acid that can help your body burn carbohydrates more efficiently for energy. This can help shore up a flagging metabolism.

1 pound boneless, skinless chicken breasts

Cilantro-Lime Dressing (page 126)

1 cup canned black beans, drained and rinsed

Pico de Gallo (page 124)

½ avocado, pitted, peeled, and chopped

¼ cup Buttermilk Ranch Dressing (page 125)

4 large butter lettuce leaves

1. In a zip-top plastic bag, combine the chicken breasts and Cilantro-Lime Dressing. Seal and refrigerate for at least 3 hours and up to overnight.

2. Preheat the oven to 425°F. Remove the chicken from the marinade and pat it dry with a paper towel. Place the chicken in a baking dish and roast for 20 to 30 minutes, or until the chicken reaches an internal temperature of 165°F. Let the chicken cool, and shred it with a fork.

3. In a medium bowl, combine the shredded chicken, beans, Pico de Gallo, avocado, and Buttermilk Ranch Dressing and mix well.

4. Spoon the mixture into the butter lettuce leaves and serve.

Tip: Save time by purchasing a precooked rotisserie chicken. Remove the meat from the bones and skin and shred it with a fork.

Per Serving: Calories: 272; Total fat: 9.5g; Saturated fat: 1.5g; Cholesterol: 63mg; Carbohydrates: 19g; Fiber: 7g; Protein: 28g

Chicken Meatball Pho

Sugar-Free

Serves 6 • **Prep time:** 15 minutes • **Cook time:** 30 minutes

Pho is a Vietnamese soup made with a fragrant broth, noodles, and beef. This lightened-up, easy version uses chicken meatballs in place of the sliced beef and zucchini noodles (zoodles) instead of rice noodles. You can buy premade zoodles in the produce section of the grocery store or hand-cut them by peeling long zucchini strips with a vegetable peeler and then using a sharp knife to cut them into noodles.

6 cups Vegetable Broth (page 130) or low-sodium chicken broth

1 star anise

2 tablespoons grated ginger, divided

6 garlic cloves, minced, divided

1 teaspoon fish sauce, divided

1 teaspoon sea salt, divided

1 pound ground chicken breast

½ cup chopped fresh cilantro, divided

2 medium zucchini, cut into zoodles

6 lime wedges, for garnish

1. In a large pot, combine the Vegetable Broth, star anise, 1 tablespoon of ginger, 3 garlic cloves, ½ teaspoon of fish sauce, and ½ teaspoon of salt and bring to a simmer over medium-high heat.

2. In a large bowl, combine the ground chicken breast, remaining 1 tablespoon of ginger, remaining 3 garlic cloves, remaining ½ teaspoon of fish sauce, remaining ½ teaspoon of salt, and ¼ cup of cilantro and mix well. Form the mixture into ½-inch meatballs.

3. Using a skimmer, remove the star anise from the simmering broth. Add the meatballs and bring the broth to a boil. Lower the heat to medium and cook until the meatballs are cooked through, about 15 minutes.

4. Add the zucchini and cook for 2 minutes more.

5. Served garnished with the lime wedges and remaining ¼ cup cilantro.

Per Serving: Calories: 103; Total fat: 1g; Saturated fat: 0g; Cholesterol: 43mg; Carbohydrates: 5g; Fiber: 1g; Protein: 19g

Turkey Taco Salad

Grain-Free, Sugar-Free

Serves 2 • **Prep time:** 10 minutes • **Cook time:** 8 minutes

When taking this for lunch, store the cooked turkey, Pico de Gallo, greens, and dressing separately and toss them together just before eating. This also makes a delicious dinner, and you can double or triple the recipe for a crowd.

1 tablespoon avocado oil

8 ounces ground turkey breast

¼ cup water

1 tablespoon chili powder

½ teaspoon ground cumin

½ teaspoon sea salt

¼ teaspoon dried oregano

4 cups mixed greens

Pico de Gallo (page 124)

¼ cup Buttermilk Ranch Dressing (page 125)

1. In a large nonstick skillet, heat the oil over medium-high heat until it shimmers.

2. Add the turkey breast and cook, crumbling it with a spoon, until browned, 5 to 7 minutes.

3. In a small bowl, whisk together the water, chili powder, cumin, salt, and oregano. Add the mixture to the skillet with the cooked meat and cook, stirring, until the meat is coated and the water evaporates, about 3 minutes.

4. In a large bowl, combine the greens, cooked turkey, and Pico de Gallo and toss until mixed.

5. Divide the mixture between two bowls and top with the Buttermilk Ranch Dressing.

Tip: You can add 2 tablespoons of shredded low-fat cheese to the salad if you wish.

Per Serving: Calories: 273; Total fat: 10g; Saturated fat: 1.5g; Cholesterol: 72mg; Carbohydrates: 18g; Fiber: 5.5g; Protein: 31g

Turkey, Veggie, and Rice Soup

Sugar-Free

Serves 6 • **Prep time:** 15 minutes • **Cook time:** 20 minutes

Soup is the perfect lunch food because you can make it ahead of time and keep it in the refrigerator or freezer for meals on the go. This will freeze for up to six months or keep in the refrigerator for up to five days. It's also a good way to use up extra vegetables, so if you have some leftover vegetables, feel free to add them.

1 tablespoon avocado oil

1 pound ground turkey breast

1 onion, chopped

2 carrots, peeled and chopped

2 celery stalks, chopped

3 garlic cloves, minced

6 cups Vegetable Broth (page 130)

1 teaspoon dried thyme

¾ teaspoon sea salt

1 cup cooked brown rice

1. In a large pot, heat the oil over medium-high heat until it shimmers.

2. Add the turkey breast and cook, crumbling it with a spoon, until it is browned, about 5 minutes.

3. Add the onion, carrots, and celery and cook, stirring occasionally, until the vegetables begin to soften, about 3 minutes.

4. Add the garlic and cook, stirring constantly, for 30 seconds.

5. Add the Vegetable Broth, thyme, and salt and bring to a simmer. Lower the heat to medium-low and simmer until the vegetables are soft, about 10 minutes. Add the rice and cook, stirring, until heated through, about 2 minutes.

Tip: Save the trimmings from your vegetables in a large zip-top plastic bag and freeze them. When the bag is full, it's time to make Vegetable Broth. It's my favorite way to reduce food waste.

Per Serving: Calories: 168; Total fat: 3.5g; Saturated fat: 0.5g; Cholesterol: 37mg; Carbohydrates: 14g; Fiber: 2g; Protein: 20g

Salmon Salad Lettuce Wraps

Grain-Free, Sugar-Free

Serves 2 • **Prep time:** 10 minutes

Skip the bread by wrapping this delicious salmon salad in tender butter lettuce. Use the large outer leaves for best results. The anise flavor of the fresh fennel complements the salmon well, and it also adds a lovely, tender crunch to these lettuce wraps.

2 (3-ounce) packages pink Pacific salmon

1 fennel bulb, cored and thinly sliced

¼ cup fresh peas (or frozen and thawed)

¼ cup plain nonfat yogurt or nondairy yogurt

1 tablespoon chopped fennel fronds (from the fennel bulb)

¼ teaspoon sea salt

⅛ teaspoon freshly ground black pepper

Grated zest and juice of ½ orange

2 large butter lettuce leaves or 4 medium leaves

1. In a medium bowl, combine the salmon, fennel bulb, and peas.

2. In a small bowl, whisk together the yogurt, fennel fronds, salt, black pepper, orange zest, and orange juice. Pour the mixture over the salmon and toss until combined.

3. Spoon the salmon mixture into the lettuce leaves and wrap them up. Serve immediately.

Tip: If you can't find fennel, replace it with chopped celery instead. You'll still get a satisfying crunch, but with a milder flavor.

Per Serving: Calories: 169; Total fat: 2.5g; Saturated fat: 0g; Cholesterol: 31mg; Carbohydrates: 16g; Fiber: 4.5g; Protein: 23g

Salmon Cobb Salad

Grain-Free

Serves 2 • **Prep time:** 15 minutes • **Cook time:** 15 minutes

If you make this ahead and take it to work, I recommend transporting the salmon and dressing in separate containers from the salad ingredients and putting it all together just before eating. The salmon will keep in an airtight container for about three days in the refrigerator, while the dressing and salad ingredients will keep for about five.

1 (6-ounce) salmon fillet, bones removed

6 tablespoons Honey-Mustard Dressing (page 127), divided

4 cups mixed greens

1 hard-boiled egg, peeled and chopped

¼ cup sliced black olives, drained and rinsed

¼ red onion, chopped

10 cherry tomatoes, halved

2 tablespoons reduced-fat blue cheese crumbles (optional)

1. Preheat the oven to 425°F.

2. Place the salmon skin-side down on a rimmed baking sheet. Brush the top with 2 tablespoons of Honey-Mustard Dressing and bake for 15 minutes, or until the salmon is opaque. Let it cool. Remove the skin and flake the fish with a fork.

3. In a large bowl, toss together the mixed greens, flaked salmon, egg, olives, onion, tomatoes, and blue cheese crumbles.

4. Add the remaining 4 tablespoons of Honey-Mustard Dressing and toss until combined. Serve immediately.

Tip: To hard-boil eggs, place them in a cold saucepan and pour in enough water to cover by 1 inch. Bring to a boil over high heat. Immediately turn off the heat (leave the pan on the burner) and cover the pot with its lid. Let the eggs sit for 14 minutes, then plunge them into ice water to stop the cooking.

Per Serving: Calories: 395; Total fat: 25g; Saturated fat: 3.5g; Cholesterol: 147mg; Carbohydrates: 18g; Fiber: 3.5g; Protein: 25g

Ginger-Lime Tuna Salad

Grain-Free, Sugar-Free

Serves 2 • **Prep time:** 10 minutes

Serve this on a bed of fresh greens or, if you wish, stuffed into a pita or as a sandwich on whole wheat bread. The tangy bite of the ginger-lime dressing is a welcome variation from a traditional mayonnaise-based tuna salad, while the water chestnuts add a nutty flavor and a fun crunch.

2 (3-ounce) packages tuna, drained and rinsed

¼ cup chopped fresh cilantro

1 (4-ounce) can sliced water chestnuts, drained and rinsed

4 scallions, green and white parts, cut into slices

2 tablespoons Ginger-Lime Marinade (page 128)

¼ cup plain nonfat yogurt

2 cups mixed greens

1. In a medium bowl, mix the tuna, cilantro, water chestnuts, and scallions.

2. In a small bowl, whisk together the Ginger-Lime Marinade and yogurt. Pour the mixture over the tuna salad and stir until combined.

3. Divide the greens equally between two plates. Spoon the tuna equally over the greens and serve.

Tip: You can replace the water chestnuts with 2 thinly sliced celery stalks or ¼ cup of fresh peas, if you wish.

Per Serving: Calories: 194; Total fat: 8g; Saturated fat: 1.5g; Cholesterol: 21mg; Carbohydrates: 17g; Fiber: 5g; Protein: 15g

Lemon-Garlic Shrimp and Orzo Salad

Sugar-Free

Serves 4 • **Prep time:** 15 minutes • **Cook time:** 10 minutes

While you can serve this right after making it, the orzo actually soaks up the liquid if you refrigerate it for a few hours, making it even more flavorful. This will keep for three days in the refrigerator, so it's easy to premake a batch and have it ready for lunch or even as a healthy dinner or side dish. With vibrant lemon, garlic, and basil flavors, it's sure to become a family favorite.

1 (16-ounce) box whole wheat or gluten-free orzo

8 ounces baby shrimp, drained and rinsed

10 basil leaves, torn

1 pint cherry tomatoes, halved

2 tablespoons extra-virgin olive oil

1 teaspoon Dijon mustard

Grated zest of ½ lemon

Juice of 2 lemons

3 garlic cloves, minced

½ teaspoon sea salt

¼ teaspoon freshly ground black pepper

1. Bring a large pot of water to a boil over high heat. Add the orzo and cook according to the package instructions. Drain the pasta and let it cool.

2. In a large bowl, toss together the cooled orzo, shrimp, basil, and tomatoes.

3. In a small bowl, whisk together the oil, mustard, lemon zest, lemon juice, garlic, salt, and black pepper. Pour the mixture over the salad and toss until combined.

Tip: Looking for a bit of heat with this salad? Add up to ½ teaspoon of red chili flakes to the dressing; add a little at a time and taste before adding more, until you achieve the desired level of heat.

Per Serving: Calories: 530; Total fat: 9.5g; Saturated fat: 1g; Cholesterol: 143mg; Carbohydrates: 83g; Fiber: 19g; Protein: 27g

Southwestern Shrimp and Avocado Salad

Grain-Free, Sugar-Free

Serves 2 • **Prep time:** 15 minutes, plus 1 hour to refrigerate

This take on ceviche uses cooked baby shrimp, so it's superfast and easy. You can choose any combination of citrus juices you wish, but a favorite of mine is equal parts freshly squeezed lemon, orange, and lime juice. This will keep in an airtight container in the refrigerator for about three days, but it doesn't freeze well.

6 ounces cooked baby shrimp

½ avocado, pitted, peeled, and chopped

¼ red onion, finely chopped

½ pint cherry tomatoes, chopped

1 jalapeño, stemmed, seeded, and minced

¼ cup chopped fresh cilantro

½ cup freshly squeezed citrus juice

1 tablespoon avocado oil

½ teaspoon sea salt

1. In a large bowl, mix the shrimp, avocado, onion, tomatoes, jalapeño, and cilantro.

2. In a smaller bowl, whisk together the citrus juice, oil, and salt. Pour the dressing over the shrimp salad and mix until combined. Cover and refrigerate for at least 1 hour and up to 8 hours before serving to allow the flavors to blend.

Tip: If you'd like to add some crunch to this salad, cut up half a peeled jicama and add it in step 2.

Per Serving: Calories: 322; Total fat: 22g; Saturated fat: 3g; Cholesterol: 123mg; Carbohydrates: 18g; Fiber: 4g; Protein: 14g

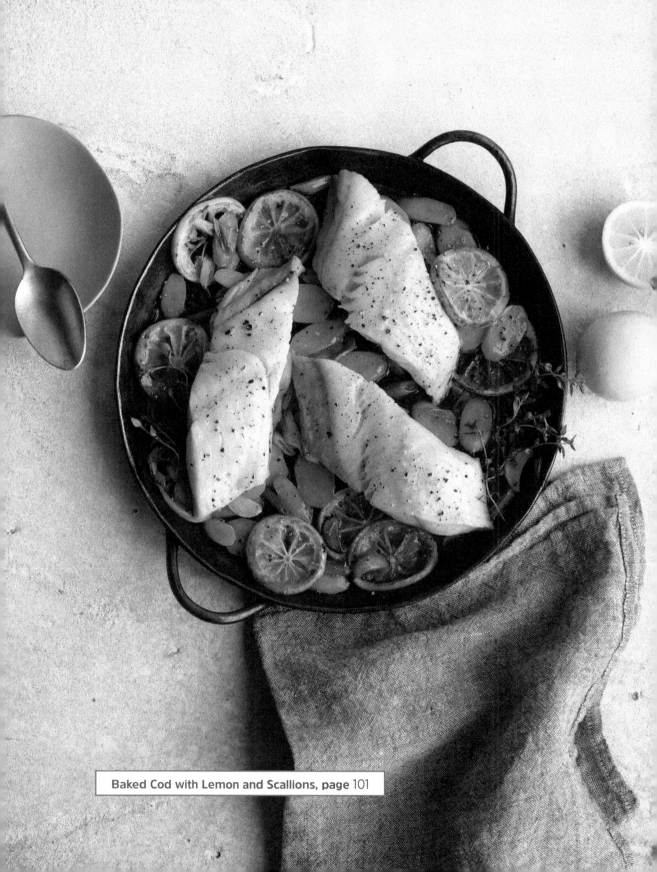

Baked Cod with Lemon and Scallions, page 101

DINNER

Vegan Pumpkin Soup

Grain-Free, Sugar-Free, Vegan

Serves 4 • **Prep time:** 10 minutes • **Cook time:** 10 minutes

Pumpkin is high in fiber and relatively low in carbohydrates, and it's loaded with antioxidants. That makes it a metabolism-boosting powerhouse, and this simple soup is a great way to showcase just how versatile and delicious pumpkin can be. Be sure to use canned unsweetened pumpkin puree and not pumpkin pie mix, which includes sugar and spices that won't work for this recipe.

1 tablespoon avocado oil

1 shallot, finely chopped

2 garlic cloves, minced

6 cups Vegetable Broth (page 130)

1 (15-ounce) can unsweetened pumpkin puree

1 teaspoon ground sage

Pinch cayenne

½ teaspoon sea salt

⅛ teaspoon freshly ground black pepper

8 tablespoons pepitas (hulled pumpkin seeds)

1. In a large pot, heat the oil over medium-high heat until it shimmers.

2. Add the shallot and cook, stirring occasionally, until soft, about 3 minutes.

3. Add the garlic and cook, stirring constantly, for 30 seconds.

4. Add the Vegetable Broth, pumpkin puree, sage, cayenne, salt, and black pepper and bring to a simmer, stirring occasionally. Lower the heat to medium and cook, stirring occasionally, for 5 minutes.

5. Spoon the soup into bowls, garnish with the pepitas, and serve.

Tip: You can also make this a butternut squash soup. In step 4, replace the pumpkin puree with 1 cubed butternut squash. Simmer the squash in the broth until it's soft, about 20 minutes. Before serving, puree the soup in a blender or food processor or with an immersion blender.

Per Serving: Calories: 193; Total fat: 11g; Saturated fat: 2g; Cholesterol: 0mg; Carbohydrates: 15g; Fiber: 4.5g; Protein: 8g

Black Bean Chili

Grain-Free, Sugar-Free, Vegan

Serves 4 • **Prep time:** 20 minutes • **Cook time:** 15 minutes

This hearty vegan chili calls on the power of black beans for fiber and protein, which makes it filling. The chili spices are also known to boost metabolism and help your body burn more calories. You can adjust the heat by using more or less cayenne.

2 tablespoons avocado oil

1 onion, chopped

1 green bell pepper, stemmed, seeded, and chopped

2 (14.5-ounce) cans crushed tomatoes, undrained

2 (15-ounce) cans black beans, drained

1 cup water

1 tablespoon chili powder

½ teaspoon ground cumin

½ teaspoon sea salt

⅛ teaspoon cayenne

1. In a large pot, heat the oil over medium-high heat until it shimmers. Add the onion and bell pepper and cook, stirring occasionally, until the vegetables are soft, about 5 minutes.

2. Add the tomatoes, beans, water, chili powder, cumin, salt, and cayenne and bring to a simmer. Lower the heat to medium-low and cook, stirring occasionally, for 10 minutes.

Tip: Want a smokier chili? Replace the chili powder with an equal amount of chipotle chili powder, which has a lovely smoked flavor.

Per Serving: Calories: 348; Total fat: 7.5g; Saturated fat: 1g; Cholesterol: 0mg; Carbohydrates: 54g; Fiber: 21g; Protein: 16g

Quick Red Beans and Rice

Sugar-Free, Vegan

Serves 4 • **Prep time:** 20 minutes • **Cook time:** 20 minutes

Both red beans and brown rice are filled with fiber, which can keep you satisfied for hours after eating it. This simple, flavorful dish calls for precooked brown rice to save you time—it's available in the rice aisle at the grocery store—or you can cook a big batch of brown rice on a weekend and freeze it in 1-cup servings for up to six months.

2 tablespoons avocado oil

1 red onion, chopped

2 celery stalks, chopped

1 green bell pepper, stemmed, seeded, and chopped

3 garlic cloves, minced

1 (15½-ounce) can small red beans, drained and rinsed

1 teaspoon smoked paprika

½ teaspoon sea salt

½ cup Vegetable Broth (page 130)

2 cups cooked brown rice

Cayenne (optional)

1. In a large nonstick skillet, heat the oil over medium-high heat until it shimmers.

2. Add the onion, celery, and bell pepper and cook, stirring occasionally, until the vegetables begin to brown, 5 to 7 minutes.

3. Add the garlic and cook, stirring constantly, for 30 seconds.

4. Add the beans, paprika, salt, and Vegetable Broth and bring to a simmer. Lower the heat to medium-low and cook, stirring occasionally, for 10 minutes.

5. Add the rice and cook, stirring, until the rice is warmed through, about 2 minutes.

6. Season with the cayenne (if using).

Tip: If desired, garnish with ¼ cup of chopped fresh parsley.

Per Serving: Calories: 298; Total fat: 8g; Saturated fat: 1g; Cholesterol: 0mg; Carbohydrates: 49g; Fiber: 9g; Protein: 9g

Black Bean Burritos

Sugar-Free, Vegan

Serves 4 • **Prep time:** 15 minutes • **Cook time:** 20 minutes

If you're a fan of Southwestern flavors, then these easy vegan burritos will hit the spot. Fragrant with cumin and chili powder, this recipe is a metabolic powerhouse thanks to the jalapeño and black beans. These burritos can be frozen for up to six months. To reheat, wrap them in aluminum foil and bake in a 350°F oven for 20 minutes.

2 tablespoons avocado oil

½ onion, finely chopped

1 green bell pepper, stemmed, seeded, and finely chopped

1 jalapeño, stemmed, seeded, and finely chopped

2 (15-ounce) cans black beans, drained

½ teaspoon sea salt

½ teaspoon ground cumin

1 tablespoon chili powder

4 (8-inch) whole wheat tortillas

Pico de Gallo (page 124)

1. Preheat the oven to 350°F. Line a rimmed baking sheet with parchment paper.

2. In a large nonstick skillet, heat the oil over medium-high heat until it shimmers. Add the onion, bell pepper, and jalapeño and cook, stirring occasionally, until the vegetables are soft and beginning to brown, 5 to 7 minutes.

3. Add the beans, salt, cumin, and chili powder and cook, stirring, until the beans are warmed through, about 5 minutes. Remove from the heat and mash with a fork or potato masher.

4. Spread the bean mixture equally on the tortillas. Wrap them up and place them on the prepared baking sheet. Bake for 20 minutes.

5. Serve topped with the Pico de Gallo.

Per Serving: Calories: 344; Total fat: 11g; Saturated fat: 1g; Cholesterol: 0mg; Carbohydrates: 57g; Fiber: 27g; Protein: 20g

Whole Wheat Pasta Puttanesca

Sugar-Free, Vegan

Serves 4 • **Prep time:** 25 minutes • **Cook time:** 20 minutes

This vegan version of puttanesca sauce is filled with boldly flavored ingredients that are richly satisfying. The heat from the red chili flakes is a well-known metabolism booster, while the beneficial fats in the black olives are also known for their anti-inflammatory and metabolism-boosting benefits.

1 (1-pound) box whole wheat farfalle (bow-tie pasta)

2 tablespoons avocado oil

1 shallot, finely chopped

4 garlic cloves, minced

2 (2½-ounce) cans sliced black olives, drained

2 tablespoons capers plus 1 tablespoon caper brine

1 (14.5-ounce) can diced tomatoes, undrained

1 tablespoon dried Italian seasoning

¼ to ½ teaspoon red chili flakes

¼ cup chopped fresh parsley

1. Bring a large pot of water to a boil over high heat. Add the pasta and cook according to the package instructions. Drain and set aside.

2. In a large nonstick skillet, heat the oil over medium-high heat until it shimmers.

3. Add the shallot and cook, stirring occasionally, until soft, about 5 minutes.

4. Add the garlic and cook, stirring constantly, for 30 seconds.

5. Add the olives, capers and caper brine, tomatoes, Italian seasoning, and red chili flakes and bring to a simmer, stirring occasionally. Lower the heat to medium-low and cook until the sauce thickens, about 5 minutes.

6. Add the pasta and cook, stirring, for 1 minute.

7. Divide the mixture onto four plates and garnish with the parsley.

Tip: If gluten is an issue, you can replace the pasta with either cooked gluten-free pasta or zucchini noodles.

Per Serving: Calories: 608; Total fat: 17g; Saturated fat: 1.5g; Cholesterol: 0mg; Carbohydrates: 103g; Fiber: 13g; Protein: 20g

Baked Chicken Tenders

Grain-Free

Serves 4 • **Prep time:** 10 minutes • **Cook time:** 30 minutes

If you're a fried chicken fan, then these quick and easy tenders are sure to please. Crusted with almond flour "bread crumbs," they're gluten-free and full of anti-inflammatory beneficial fats from the almonds. Serve them with a simple side salad for a full meal.

½ cup almond flour

1 teaspoon garlic powder

1 teaspoon dried thyme

½ teaspoon sea salt

¼ teaspoon freshly ground black pepper

2 eggs, beaten

1 tablespoon Dijon mustard

1 pound chicken breast tenders

Honey-Mustard Dressing (page 127)

1. Preheat the oven to 425°F.

2. In a shallow dish, whisk together the almond flour, garlic powder, thyme, salt, and black pepper. Set aside.

3. In a medium bowl, whisk together the eggs and mustard.

4. Dip each tender in the egg mixture and then in the flour mixture, tapping off any excess flour, and place on a rimmed nonstick baking sheet.

5. Bake for 25 to 30 minutes, or until the chicken reaches an internal temperature of 165°F.

6. Serve with the Honey-Mustard Dressing as a dipping sauce.

Tip: Almond flour can be found in the baking aisle of most grocery stores, but if you can't find it, you can make your own easily if you have a food processor. Simply pulse blanched almonds in the food processor in 1-second pulses 10 to 20 times, until they reach the desired consistency.

Per Serving: Calories: 336; Total fat: 16g; Saturated fat: 2.5g; Cholesterol: 146mg; Carbohydrates: 13g; Fiber: 1g; Protein: 29g

Turkey Burgers

Sugar-Free

Serves 4 • **Prep time:** 10 minutes • **Cook time:** 10 minutes

Lighten up burger night with these delicious turkey burgers that feature Spicy Secret Sauce. Adding fish sauce to the ground turkey may sound odd, but it adds a savory element to the patties that gives them a deeper flavor.

1 pound ground turkey breast

1 teaspoon fish sauce

2 garlic cloves, minced

½ teaspoon red chili flakes

½ teaspoon sea salt

1 tablespoon avocado oil

4 whole wheat hamburger buns, toasted

4 lettuce leaves

4 tomato slices

Spicy Secret Sauce (page 123)

1. In a large bowl, mix the ground turkey, fish sauce, garlic, red chili flakes, and salt and form the mixture into 4 patties.

2. In a large nonstick skillet, heat the oil over medium-high heat until it shimmers, swirling to coat the pan.

3. Add the patties and cook until they are browned and reach an internal temperature of 165°F, about 5 minutes per side.

4. Place a burger on each of the bottom buns and top each with a lettuce leaf, a tomato slice, and 2 tablespoons of Spicy Secret Sauce. Place the remaining buns on top and serve.

Tip: Unsure about fish sauce? You can replace it with an equal amount of either Worcestershire sauce or reduced-sodium soy sauce, but omit the salt if you do.

Per Serving: Calories: 350; Total fat: 8.5g; Saturated fat: 1.5g; Cholesterol: 73mg; Carbohydrates: 34g; Fiber: 8g; Protein: 38g

Turkey Sloppy Joes

Serves 4 • **Prep time:** 15 minutes • **Cook time:** 20 minutes

There's a reason sloppy joes are a family favorite; they're tangy and delicious and easy to make. This lightened-up version replaces ground beef with lean ground turkey breast, but it doesn't sacrifice flavor. You can lighten these sloppy joes up even further by replacing the buns with lettuce cups as a serving vessel or spooning the sauce into whole-grain pitas.

2 tablespoons avocado oil

1 pound ground turkey breast

1 onion, finely chopped

1 green bell pepper, stemmed, seeded, and finely chopped

3 garlic cloves, minced

¼ cup apple cider vinegar

1 (15-ounce) can crushed tomatoes

1 teaspoon chili powder

½ teaspoon Worcestershire sauce

4 whole wheat hamburger buns

1. In a large nonstick skillet, heat the oil over medium-high heat until it shimmers. Add the turkey breast and cook, crumbling it with a spoon, until browned, about 5 minutes.

2. Add the onion and bell pepper and cook, stirring occasionally, until soft, about 4 minutes more.

3. Add the garlic and cook, stirring constantly, for 30 seconds.

4. Add the vinegar and stir, using the spoon to scrape any browned bits from the bottom of the pan. Add the tomatoes, chili powder, and Worcestershire sauce and bring to a simmer. Lower the heat to medium and cook, stirring occasionally, until the sauce is thick, about 3 minutes.

5. Serve spooned over the buns.

Tip: Make these vegan by replacing the ground turkey breast with a 15-ounce can of cooked lentils, drained.

Per Serving: Calories: 386; Total fat: 11g; Saturated fat: 2g; Cholesterol: 72mg; Carbohydrates: 35g; Fiber: 6.5g; Protein: 30g

Tex-Mex Turkey Meatballs

Sugar-Free

Serves 4 • **Prep time:** 20 minutes • **Cook time:** 30 minutes

These meatballs are simmered in a spicy red sauce and then served over cooked brown rice. The spices can help boost metabolism, while the protein in the turkey and the fiber in the rice are filling and satisfying. These freeze well for up to six months, so feel free to mix up a double batch for lunches.

2 tablespoons avocado oil, divided

1 onion, chopped

1 jalapeño, stemmed, seeded, and finely chopped

1 pound ground turkey breast

3 teaspoons chili powder, divided

1 teaspoon sea salt, divided

1 teaspoon garlic powder, divided

1 (15-ounce) can crushed tomatoes, undrained

1 (10-ounce) can diced tomatoes and green chiles, drained

4 cups cooked brown rice

1. In a large nonstick skillet, heat 1 tablespoon of oil over medium-high heat until it shimmers. Add the onion and jalapeño and cook, stirring occasionally, until soft, about 4 minutes. Let cool.

2. In a bowl, mix the ground turkey, cooled onion and jalapeño, 2 teaspoons of chili powder, ½ teaspoon of salt, and ½ teaspoon of garlic powder. Form the mixture into ½-inch meatballs. Set them aside on a plate.

3. In the same pan you used to cook the onion and jalapeño, heat the remaining 1 tablespoon of oil over medium-high heat until it shimmers. Add the meatballs and cook, turning them occasionally, until browned, about 10 minutes. Remove from the pan and set aside on the plate.

4. Add the crushed tomatoes, diced tomatoes and chiles, remaining 1 teaspoon of chili powder, remaining ½ teaspoon of salt, and remaining ½ teaspoon of garlic powder to the same pan and bring to a boil, stirring frequently. Lower the heat to medium, add the meatballs, and cook, covered, turning the meatballs occasionally, until they reach an internal temperature of 165°F, about 10 minutes.

5. Serve the meatballs and sauce spooned over the cooked rice.

Tip: You can also make these in a slow cooker. Place the uncooked meatballs in a slow cooker with all the other ingredients except the cooked rice. Cover and cook on low for 8 hours. Spoon the meatballs and sauce over the cooked rice.

Per Serving: Calories: 508; Total fat: 11g; Saturated fat: 2g; Cholesterol: 72mg; Carbohydrates: 65g; Fiber: 7g; Protein: 35g

Ground Turkey and Cauliflower Rice Stir-Fry

Grain-Free, Sugar-Free

Serves 4 • **Prep time:** 20 minutes • **Cook time:** 15 minutes

Cauliflower rice is a nutritious, grain-free substitute for rice that cooks more quickly and is loaded with fiber and nutrients that will boost your metabolism. You can purchase it in the rice aisle of the grocery store premade or save money by making your own. Simply grate cauliflower on a box grater to make rice.

2 tablespoons avocado oil

12 ounces ground turkey breast

8 scallions, white and green parts, chopped

2 cups broccoli florets

1 red bell pepper, stemmed, seeded, and chopped

1 cup shredded cabbage

2 cups cauliflower rice

Ginger-Lime Marinade (page 128)

¼ cup chopped fresh cilantro

2 tablespoons sesame seeds

1. In a large nonstick skillet, heat the oil over medium-high heat until it shimmers. Add the turkey and cook, crumbling it with a spoon, until browned, about 5 minutes.

2. Using a slotted spoon, transfer the turkey to a bowl and set it aside.

3. Add the scallions, broccoli, bell pepper, and cabbage to the pan and cook, stirring, until crisp-tender, about 5 minutes.

4. Add the cauliflower rice and Ginger-Lime Marinade and cook, stirring, until the cauliflower is tender, about 4 minutes. Put the cooked turkey back in the pan, stir to combine, and heat through.

5. Serve garnished with the cilantro and sesame seeds.

Tip: If you have a food processor, making cauliflower rice is superfast. Simply break a head of cauliflower into florets, put it in your food processor fitted with a chopping blade, and pulse in 1-second bursts 10 to 20 times, until it resembles rice.

Per Serving: Calories: 309; Total fat: 18g; Saturated fat: 2.5g; Cholesterol: 54mg; Carbohydrates: 12g; Fiber: 4.5g; Protein: 25g

Hand-Cut Zoodles with Turkey Bolognese

Grain-Free, Sugar-Free

Serves 4 • **Prep time:** 20 minutes • **Cook time:** 20 minutes

A simple ground turkey Bolognese, like this one, can also be made vegan by replacing the ground turkey with either chopped extra-firm tofu, diced mushrooms, or tempeh. The tomato sauce is full of lycopene, an antioxidant that can help reduce inflammation, as well as aromatic spices that can boost metabolism.

2 tablespoons avocado oil, divided

1 pound ground turkey breast

1 onion, finely chopped

1 red bell pepper, stemmed, seeded, and chopped

4 garlic cloves, minced

1 (28-ounce) can crushed tomatoes with basil and oregano, drained

1 tablespoon dried Italian seasoning

¼ teaspoon red chili flakes

½ teaspoon sea salt

4 medium zucchini, cut into noodles

1. In a large nonstick skillet, heat 1 tablespoon of oil over medium-high heat until it shimmers. Add the turkey and cook, crumbling it with a spoon, until browned, about 5 minutes. Transfer the turkey to a plate and set it aside.

2. In the same pan, heat the remaining 1 tablespoon of oil over medium-high heat until it shimmers. Add the onion and bell pepper and cook, stirring occasionally, until soft, about 5 minutes.

3. Add the garlic and cook, stirring constantly, for 30 seconds.

4. Add the tomatoes, Italian seasoning, red chili flakes, salt, and cooked turkey and bring to a simmer. Lower the heat to medium-low and cook, stirring occasionally, for 5 minutes more.

5. Add the zucchini and cook, stirring occasionally, for 5 minutes.

Tip: Add even more fresh flavor by garnishing each serving with 2 tablespoons of chopped fresh basil.

Per Serving: Calories: 316; Total fat: 9g; Saturated fat: 1.5g; Cholesterol: 55mg; Carbohydrates: 27g; Fiber: 6g; Protein: 33g

Mustard Roasted Pork Tenderloin and Sweet Potatoes

Grain-Free

Serves 4 • **Prep time:** 20 minutes, plus 4 hours to marinate
Cook time: 40 minutes

Pork tenderloin is a good source of lean protein. Sweet potatoes are high in antioxidants and metabolism-boosting fiber.

Honey-Mustard
   Dressing (page 127),
   divided

1 (1-pound) pork
   tenderloin

4 sweet potatoes,
   peeled and cut into
   ½-inch pieces

8 shallots, peeled and
   quartered

1 tablespoon avocado
   oil

1 teaspoon dried thyme

½ teaspoon sea salt

¼ teaspoon freshly
   ground black pepper

1. In a large zip-top plastic bag, combine all but 2 tablespoons of the Honey-Mustard Dressing with the tenderloin. Seal and refrigerate for at least 4 hours and up to 12 hours.

2. Preheat the oven to 400°F.

3. Remove the tenderloin from the marinade and pat it dry with paper towels. Place it in a roasting pan or baking dish. Set aside.

4. In a medium bowl, toss the sweet potatoes and shallots with the oil, thyme, salt, and black pepper. Arrange the mixture in the roasting pan around the tenderloin.

5. Bake for 40 minutes, or until the potatoes are tender and the tenderloin reaches an internal temperature of 145°F.

6. Tent the tenderloin with aluminum foil and let it rest for 10 minutes. Cut the tenderloin into four slices. Toss the potatoes and shallots with the remaining 2 tablespoons of Honey-Mustard Dressing. Divide the tenderloin and potatoes among four plates and serve.

Tip: Replace the sweet potatoes with 4 cups of cubed winter squash for a sweet and earthy variation.

Per Serving: Calories: 434; Total fat: 13g; Saturated fat: 2g; Cholesterol: 74mg; Carbohydrates: 49g; Fiber: 6.5g; Protein: 28g

Citrus-Soy Salmon and Veggie Packets

Grain-Free, Sugar-Free

Serves 4 • **Prep time:** 20 minutes • **Cook time:** 30 minutes

Salmon is a good source of anti-inflammatory omega-3 fatty acids, and it's also an excellent source of lean protein. Select wild-caught Pacific salmon, which has a much higher concentration of omega-3s and is therefore more nutritious than Atlantic or farmed salmon.

Citrus-Soy Marinade
(page 129)

½ teaspoon sesame oil

4 (4-ounce) salmon
fillets

4 cups sliced summer
squash, such as
zucchini or pattypan
squash

1 onion, thinly sliced

1. In a shallow dish, whisk together the Citrus-Soy Marinade and sesame oil.

2. Place the salmon fillets in the dish, skin-side up, and let rest for about 10 minutes.

3. Preheat the oven to 375°F. Cut four 12-by-12-inch squares of aluminum foil.

4. Remove the salmon from the marinade and pat it dry with paper towels. Place one fillet on each square of foil.

5. Top with the squash and onion and fold the foil into packets. Place the packets on a rimmed baking sheet.

6. Bake for 30 minutes, or until the vegetables are soft and the salmon is opaque.

Tip: No need to peel the squash before you cut it. The peel is edible and adds texture and color as well as fiber and nutrients to the dish.

Per Serving: Calories: 249; Total fat: 13g; Saturated fat: 2g; Cholesterol: 62mg; Carbohydrates: 9g; Fiber: 2g; Protein: 25g

Cod Piccata with Zoodles

Grain-Free, Sugar-Free

Serves 4 • **Prep time:** 10 minutes • **Cook time:** 15 minutes

Cod is an excellent source of anti-inflammatory beneficial omega-3 fatty acids, and it's low in fat and calories while still offering satisfying protein. When combined with a tangy piccata sauce and served atop a bed of zucchini noodles, it's the perfect fast weeknight supper.

¼ cup almond flour

½ teaspoon sea salt

4 (4-ounce) cod fillets, bones and skin removed

2 tablespoons avocado oil

1 shallot, finely chopped

2 garlic cloves, minced

Grated zest of 1 lemon

Juice of 2 lemons

2 tablespoons capers, drained and rinsed

4 medium zucchini, cut into noodles

¼ cup chopped fresh parsley

1. In a shallow dish, whisk together the almond flour and salt.

2. Dip the cod pieces into the almond flour mixture until completely coated and tap away any excess flour. Place on a plate.

3. In a large nonstick skillet, heat the oil over medium-high heat until it shimmers.

4. Add the cod and cook until browned, about 4 minutes per side. Transfer the cod to another plate and set aside.

5. Add the shallot and garlic to the pan and cook, stirring, for 1 minute.

6. Add the lemon zest and lemon juice and stir, using the spoon to scrape any browned bits from the bottom of the pan. Add the capers and cook, stirring, until the liquid reduces by half, about 5 minutes.

7. Add the zucchini noodles to the pan and cook, stirring, for 5 minutes.

8. Remove from the heat, stir in the parsley, and divide between four plates. Serve hot, topped with the cod.

Tip: You can also make this dish with turkey breast fillets. Pound the breast fillets to a ¼-inch thickness before cooking for about 2 minutes per side. Proceed with the recipe as written.

Per Serving: Calories: 222; Total fat: 11g; Saturated fat: 1.5g; Cholesterol: 43mg; Carbohydrates: 10g; Fiber: 3g; Protein: 22g

Ginger-Lime Cod Tacos

Grain-Free, Sugar-Free

Serves 4 • **Prep time:** 20 minutes • **Cook time:** 15 minutes

These tacos use tender butter lettuce in place of taco shells, which reduces the calories and adds nutrients. They're also anti-inflammatory thanks to the presence of ginger, which adds a pleasing heat to these yummy wraps.

Cilantro-Lime Dressing (page 126)

1 tablespoon grated ginger

1 pound cod, skin and bones removed, cut into 1-inch cubes

1 tablespoon avocado oil

2 cups coleslaw mix

¼ cup chopped fresh cilantro

8 scallions, white and green parts, thinly sliced

8 large butter lettuce leaves

1. In a small bowl, whisk together the Cilantro-Lime Dressing and ginger. Reserve 2 tablespoons and combine the rest with the cod in a zip-top plastic bag. Seal and refrigerate for 10 minutes.

2. Remove the cod from the marinade and pat it dry with paper towels.

3. In a large nonstick skillet, heat the oil over medium-high heat until it shimmers. Add the cod and cook, stirring, until it's opaque, about 10 minutes.

4. In a medium bowl, toss together the coleslaw mix, cilantro, scallions, and reserved 2 tablespoons of marinade.

5. Assemble the tacos by dividing the cooked cod between 8 lettuce leaves and topping with the slaw. Wrap up each lettuce leaf and serve.

Per Serving: Calories: 232; Total fat: 15g; Saturated fat: 2g; Cholesterol: 43mg; Carbohydrates: 5g; Fiber: 1g; Protein: 19g

Baked Cod with Lemon and Scallions

Grain-Free, Sugar-Free

Serves 4 • **Prep time:** 10 minutes • **Cook time:** 15 minutes

Cod works well in fish recipes because it's so easy to find either in the fresh fish section or in the freezer section of the grocery store. Feel free to substitute an equal amount of any white-fleshed fish, such as halibut or snapper—whatever is available locally for you.

2 tablespoons avocado oil, divided

2 small carrots, peeled and thinly sliced

2 scallions, white and green parts, cut into ½-inch pieces

1 garlic clove, thinly sliced

1 lemon, thinly sliced

1 teaspoon sea salt, divided

4 (4-ounce) skinless cod fillets

¼ teaspoon freshly ground black pepper

4 thyme sprigs

1. Preheat the oven to 400°F.

2. In a large ovenproof skillet, heat 1 tablespoon of oil over medium-high heat until it shimmers.

3. Add the carrots and cook, stirring occasionally, until they begin to soften, about 5 minutes.

4. Remove from the heat and add the scallions, garlic, and lemon slices. Season with ½ teaspoon of salt and stir to coat the ingredients with the oil in the pan.

5. Arrange the cod on top of the vegetables. Drizzle with the remaining 1 tablespoon of oil and sprinkle with the remaining ½ teaspoon of salt and the black pepper. Top with the thyme sprigs.

6. Bake until the cod is opaque, about 15 minutes.

7. Divide the cod and vegetables between four plates and serve.

Tip: You can enjoy this as is or serve it with ½ cup of cooked cauliflower rice per serving for a hearty, grain-free meal.

Per Serving: Calories: 158; Total fat: 8g; Saturated fat: 1g; Cholesterol: 43mg; Carbohydrates: 3g; Fiber: 1g; Protein: 18g

Easy Corn and Shrimp Chowder

Sugar-Free

Serves 4 • **Prep time:** 20 minutes • **Cook time:** 30 minutes

Shrimp and corn have a natural affinity in this delicious chowder, which is loaded with satiating fiber and satisfying flavor. This freezes well for up to six months, so it's easy to double the batch for extra lunchtime meals on the run during the week.

2 tablespoons avocado oil

1 onion, chopped

1 fennel bulb, chopped

1 red bell pepper, stemmed, seeded, and chopped

2 tablespoons all-purpose flour

6 cups Vegetable Broth (page 130)

½ teaspoon sea salt

¼ teaspoon freshly ground black pepper

1 (11-ounce) can corn kernels (preferably summer corn), drained

12 ounces cooked baby shrimp

1 tablespoon chopped fennel fronds (from the fennel bulb)

1. In a large pot, heat the oil over medium-high heat until it shimmers. Add the onion, fennel bulb, and bell pepper and cook, stirring occasionally, until the vegetables are soft, about 5 minutes.

2. Add the flour and cook, stirring constantly, for about 1 minute.

3. Add the Vegetable Broth, salt, and black pepper and cook, stirring occasionally, until the chowder comes to a boil and begins to thicken.

4. Stir in the corn, shrimp, and fennel fronds and cook, stirring, for 1 minute. Spoon into bowls and serve.

Tip: If you're allergic to shellfish, this chowder can easily be adapted for another type of fish, such as salmon or cod. Simply replace the cooked shrimp with 12 ounces of chopped fish and allow it to cook in the soup for about 5 minutes, until the fish is opaque.

Per Serving: Calories: 342; Total fat: 18g; Saturated fat: 2.5g; Cholesterol: 123mg; Carbohydrates: 31g; Fiber: 5g; Protein: 16g

Shrimp Scampi

Grain-Free, Sugar-Free

Serves 4 • **Prep time:** 20 minutes • **Cook time:** 15 minutes

This garlic-scented scampi uses zucchini noodles in place of grain-based noodles, so it's a lighter version that's still delicious. To make zucchini noodles, simply cut them into long strips with a vegetable peeler and then use a sharp knife to cut them to the desired width.

2 tablespoons avocado oil

1 shallot, finely minced

12 ounces medium shrimp, peeled, deveined, and tails removed

6 garlic cloves, minced

Grated zest of 1 lemon

Juice of 2 lemons

½ teaspoon sea salt

⅛ teaspoon freshly ground black pepper

Pinch red chili flakes

2 medium zucchini, cut into noodles

1. In a large skillet, heat the oil over medium-high heat until it shimmers. Add the shallot and cook, stirring occasionally, until soft, about 4 minutes.

2. Add the shrimp and cook, stirring, until opaque, about 4 minutes.

3. Add the garlic and cook, stirring constantly, for 30 seconds.

4. Add the lemon zest, lemon juice, salt, black pepper, and red chili flakes and cook, stirring, for 2 minutes.

5. Add the zucchini noodles and cook, stirring occasionally, for 5 minutes more. Serve immediately.

Tip: Devein shrimp under running water by cutting along the spine with a sharp paring knife and using the tip of the knife to remove the vein.

Per Serving: Calories: 157; Total fat: 8g; Saturated fat: 1g; Cholesterol: 119mg; Carbohydrates: 7g; Fiber: 1.5g; Protein: 17g

Grilled Shrimp with Mango-Cucumber Salsa

Grain-Free, Sugar-Free

Serves 4 • **Prep time:** 10 minutes, plus 30 minutes to marinate
Cook time: 30 minutes

Cook these shrimp on any grill—indoor or outdoor—or even using a plug-in grill or a stovetop grill pan. Be sure to soak wooden skewers for about 1 hour in fresh water before threading your shrimp to prevent them from catching fire.

Cilantro-Lime Dressing
(page 126)

1 pound large shrimp,
peeled and deveined

2 tablespoons
avocado oil,
divided

1 large mango, peeled,
pitted, and cubed

1 small cucumber,
diced

1 scallion, green and
white parts, thinly
sliced

1 tablespoon freshly
squeezed lime juice

¼ teaspoon sea salt

1. In a zip-top plastic bag, combine the Cilantro-Lime Dressing and shrimp. Seal and refrigerate for 30 minutes.

2. Remove the shrimp from the marinade and pat them dry with a paper towel. Thread the shrimp on skewers, about two shrimp per skewer.

3. Heat a grill pan or grill over high heat. Brush with 1 tablespoon of oil.

4. Grill the skewers until the shrimp are opaque, 3 to 4 minutes per side.

5. While the shrimp cooks, in a bowl combine the mango, cucumber, scallion, lime juice, remaining 1 tablespoon of oil, and salt and mix well.

6. Spoon the mango-cucumber salsa over the shrimp skewers and serve.

Tip: To cut a mango, use a sharp knife to cut lengthwise, running the knife along the edges of the pit so you get two slices with the fruit and skin and one center piece with the pit. Cut each slice with fruit and skin in a grid pattern through the flesh until you reach the skin, but without cutting through the skin. With a spoon, scoop out the cubed flesh.

Per Serving: Calories: 235; Total fat: 11g; Saturated fat: 1.5g; Cholesterol: 159mg; Carbohydrates: 14g; Fiber: 1.5g; Protein: 21g

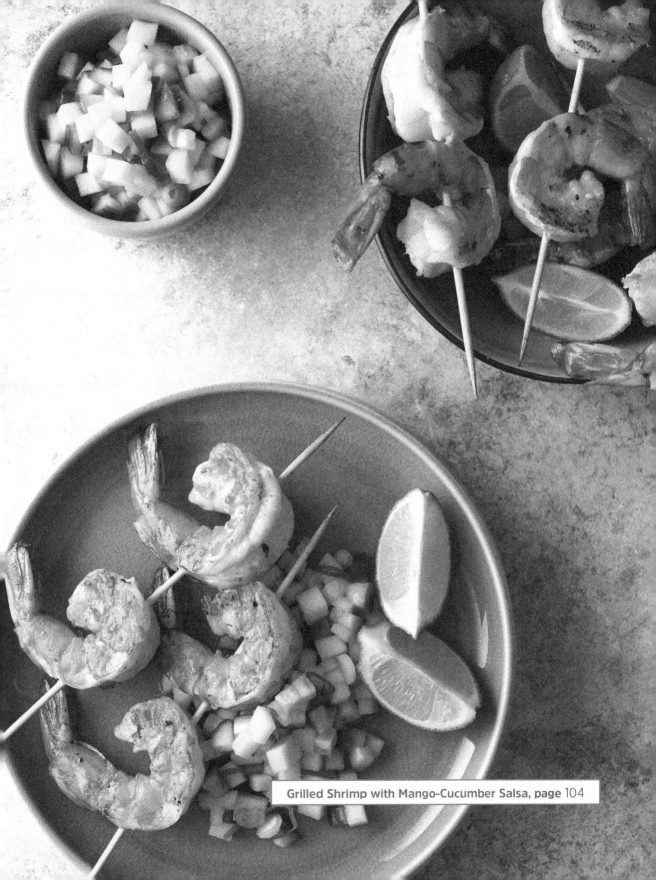

Grilled Shrimp with Mango-Cucumber Salsa, page 104

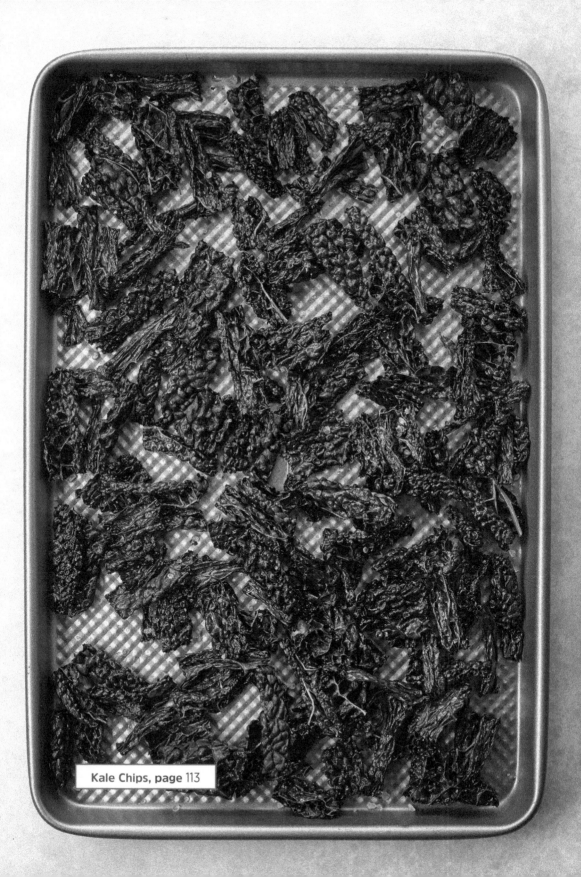
Kale Chips, page 113

SNACKS

Hummus

Grain-Free, Sugar-Free, Vegan

Makes 1¼ cups • **Prep time:** 20 minutes

Smooth and creamy, hummus is packed with flavor and nutrition. Extra-virgin olive oil adds beneficial, anti-inflammatory fats, while the chickpeas are loaded with fiber. Sliced red bell peppers for dipping add an element of crispy sweetness that makes this the perfect well-balanced snack.

1 (15-ounce) can chickpeas, drained

2 tablespoons tahini

2 garlic cloves, minced

Juice of 1 lemon

½ teaspoon ground turmeric

2 tablespoons extra-virgin olive oil

½ teaspoon sea salt

2 red bell peppers (optional), stemmed, seeded, and cut into sticks, for serving

1. In a blender or food processor, combine the chickpeas, tahini, garlic, lemon juice, turmeric, oil, and salt and blend until smooth.

2. If desired, serve with the bell peppers for dipping.

Tip: Just about any crispy veggie tastes good dipped in hummus. Try it with sliced carrots, cherry tomatoes, celery sticks, or sliced radishes.

Per Serving (¼ cup): Calories: 158; Total fat: 10g; Saturated fat: 1.5g; Cholesterol: 0mg; Carbohydrates: 14g; Fiber: 3.5g; Protein: 5g

Fiesta Corn Salad

Sugar-Free, Vegan

Serves 4 • **Prep time:** 10 minutes, plus 30 minutes to refrigerate

While many people consider corn a vegetable, it's actually a grain, and it's especially high in fiber, so it keeps you feeling full long after you eat it. This salad works best with corn cut fresh from the cob, but if corn isn't in season, you can also use canned summer corn that has been drained.

1½ cups sweet corn kernels

½ cup canned black beans, drained

1 red bell pepper, stemmed, seeded, and finely chopped

½ red onion, finely chopped

1 garlic clove, minced

1 tomato, diced

¼ cup chopped fresh cilantro

Cilantro-Lime Dressing (page 126)

1. In a large bowl, mix the corn, beans, bell pepper, onion, garlic, tomato, and cilantro.

2. Add the Cilantro-Lime Dressing and toss until combined. Cover with plastic wrap and refrigerate for at least 30 minutes or up to 1 day before serving.

Tip: The longer you allow this to rest in the refrigerator, the better the flavors combine, so it's a good make-ahead recipe.

Per Serving: Calories: 222; Total fat: 15g; Saturated fat: 2g; Cholesterol: 0mg; Carbohydrates: 21g; Fiber: 4.5g; Protein: 4g

Guacamole

Grain-Free, Sugar-Free, Vegan

Makes ½ cup • **Prep time:** 10 minutes

Jicama is a crisp root vegetable with a slight bite that's a perfect stand-in for chips. It can usually be found in the produce section of the grocery store, but if you can't find it, feel free to replace it with sliced carrots, sliced bell peppers, or cherry tomatoes for dipping. Guacamole also makes a delicious sandwich spread, and it's terrific on burgers.

1 avocado, pitted, peeled, and cubed

Juice of ½ lime

¼ red onion, finely chopped

1 garlic clove, minced

2 tablespoons chopped fresh cilantro

¼ teaspoon sea salt

1 jicama (optional), peeled and sliced, for serving

1. Place the avocado in a medium bowl and squeeze the lime juice over the top. Add the onion, garlic, cilantro, and salt and mash with a fork until combined.

2. If desired, serve with the jicama slices for dipping.

Tip: Guacamole oxidizes quickly, even when you refrigerate it, which results in a brown color and off flavors. You can counter this by placing plastic wrap directly on the surface of the guacamole and storing it in the refrigerator, which keeps oxygen out and slows the oxidation reaction.

Per Serving (2 tablespoons guacamole): Calories: 61; Total fat: 5g; Saturated fat: 0.5g; Cholesterol: 0mg; Carbohydrates: 4g; Fiber: 2.5g; Protein: 1g

Per Serving (2 tablespoons guacamole + jicama): Calories: 123; Total fat: 5.5g; Saturated fat: 0.5g; Cholesterol: 0mg; Carbohydrates: 18g; Fiber: 11g; Protein: 2g

Spicy Bean Dip

Grain-Free, Sugar-Free, Vegan

Serves 6 • **Prep time:** 10 minutes

This is another dip that tastes good no matter what you dip in it. Enjoy it with baked tortilla chips, sliced jicama, or your favorite sliced vegetables, or spread it on a corn tortilla or in a whole wheat pita half for a delicious, high-fiber snack.

1 (15-ounce) can pinto beans, drained

½ jalapeño, stemmed, seeded, and finely minced

Juice of 1 lime

¼ red onion, finely minced

2 garlic cloves, minced

½ teaspoon chipotle chili powder

Pinch cayenne

½ teaspoon sea salt

2 to 4 tablespoons water

Pico de Gallo (page 124)

1. In a blender or food processor, combine the beans, jalapeño, lime juice, onion, garlic, chili powder, cayenne, and salt and blend until smooth, adding water by the tablespoon to reach the desired consistency. Taste and add more cayenne until the mixture is as spicy as you like it.

2. Transfer the bean mixture to a bowl and fold in the Pico de Gallo.

3. Serve as a spread or dip.

Per Serving: Calories: 78; Total fat: 0.5g; Saturated fat: 0g; Cholesterol: 0mg; Carbohydrates: 15g; Fiber: 4.5g; Protein: 4g

Hummus Deviled Eggs

Grain-Free, Sugar-Free

Serves 6 • **Prep time:** 10 minutes

Hummus serves as a lower-fat stand-in for mayonnaise in these tasty deviled eggs. This adds tremendous flavor while keeping the filling smooth and appealing. You can use the traditional Hummus (page 108) in this chapter or the Beet Hummus (page 122) in the Staples chapter.

6 hard-boiled eggs, peeled and halved lengthwise

½ cup Hummus or Beet Hummus

Dash sugar-free hot sauce

¼ cup chopped fresh basil

1. Scoop the yolks from the egg halves and put them in a medium bowl. Place the egg whites cut-side up on a serving platter.

2. Add the Hummus, hot sauce, and basil to the bowl with the yolks and mash them with a fork. Add more hot sauce as desired.

3. Spoon the filling into the egg whites and serve.

Per Serving: Calories: 138; Total fat: 9g; Saturated fat: 2g; Cholesterol: 186mg; Carbohydrates: 6g; Fiber: 1.5g; Protein: 8g

Kale Chips

Grain-Free, Sugar-Free, Vegan

Serves 4 • **Prep time:** 10 minutes • **Cook time:** 30 minutes

Kale chips don't take much active time, although it does take some patience to wait until they get nice and crispy in the oven. The trick to getting them crispy is to use paper towels to pat the kale completely dry before baking the chips. Kale is full of fiber and beneficial vitamins and antioxidants, making these the perfect metabolism-boosting snack.

1 large bunch kale, washed, dried, and ribs removed, cut into 2-inch pieces

2 tablespoons avocado oil

1 teaspoon sea salt

1. Preheat the oven to 275°F. Line two rimmed baking sheets with parchment paper.

2. In a large bowl, toss the kale with the oil and salt. Spread out the kale in a single layer on the baking sheets.

3. Bake for 15 minutes. Flip the kale and bake for another 15 minutes, or until crisp.

Tip: To flavor the kale chips, you can add ¼ teaspoon of garlic powder with the sea salt, or you can replace 1 teaspoon of the avocado oil with sesame oil or chili oil. For a cheesy kale chip, toss the baked chips with 1 tablespoon of nutritional yeast before cooling.

Per Serving: Calories: 102; Total fat: 8g; Saturated fat: 1g; Cholesterol: 0mg; Carbohydrates: 7g; Fiber: 3g; Protein: 3g

Rosemary Sweet Potato Chips

Grain-Free, Sugar-Free, Vegan

Serves 4 • **Prep time:** 10 minutes • **Cook time:** 30 minutes

The trick to crisp baked chips is to cut them into the thinnest slices you can. This is easily accomplished with an extremely sharp knife, by using the slicing side of a box grater, by cutting with a vegetable peeler, or by using a mandoline. Try to cut the chips to a thickness of about ⅛ inch for best results.

2 sweet potatoes, cut into ⅛-inch-thick slices

2 tablespoons avocado oil

2 tablespoons chopped fresh rosemary

½ teaspoon sea salt

1. Preheat the oven to 350°F. Line two rimmed baking sheets with parchment paper.

2. In a large bowl, toss together the sweet potato slices, oil, rosemary, and salt. Spread the sweet potato slices out in a single layer on the baking sheets.

3. Bake for 15 minutes. Flip the sweet potato slices and bake for about 10 minutes more, or until crisp. Let cool.

Tip: You can make chips from other root vegetables, such as potatoes or carrots, using the same recipe and method.

Per Serving: Calories: 118; Total fat: 7g; Saturated fat: 1g; Cholesterol: 0mg; Carbohydrates: 13g; Fiber: 2g; Protein: 1g

Pear and Walnut Salad

Grain-Free, Vegan

Serves 4 • **Prep time:** 10 minutes

Pears have a sweet, mellow flavor that's perfect when combined with crunchy, nutritious walnuts. Along with the healthy fats in the walnuts, the pears have fiber and the ginger is anti-inflammatory, making this salad a great, metabolism-boosting pick-me-up.

4 pears, peeled, cored, and cut into ½-inch pieces

¼ cup dried cranberries

¼ cup chopped walnuts

1 tablespoon grated fresh ginger

Juice of 1 lemon

1 tablespoon avocado oil

1. In a large bowl, mix the pears, cranberries, and walnuts.

2. In a small bowl, whisk together the ginger, lemon juice, and oil. Add the ginger mixture to the pears and toss until combined.

Tip: Replace the walnuts with Pumpkin Spice Pepitas (page 116) for a tasty variation on this salad.

Per Serving: Calories: 203; Total fat: 8.5g; Saturated fat: 1g; Cholesterol: 0mg; Carbohydrates: 34g; Fiber: 6.5g; Protein: 2g

Pumpkin Spice Pepitas

Grain-Free, Vegan

Serves 6 • **Prep time:** 5 minutes • **Cook time:** 25 minutes

Pepitas are hulled pumpkin seeds and have a lovely flavor that works well with both sweet and savory spices. They're loaded with vitamins and beneficial fats, and they are a satisfying snack when you're trying to boost your metabolism.

¾ cup raw pepitas (hulled pumpkin seeds)

2 tablespoons avocado oil

2 tablespoons Pumpkin Pie Spice Blend (page 131)

1 tablespoon pure maple syrup

1. Preheat the oven to 350°F. Line a rimmed baking sheet with parchment paper.

2. In a small bowl, combine the pepitas, oil, Pumpkin Pie Spice Blend, and maple syrup and mix well. Spread the pepitas in a single layer on the prepared baking sheet.

3. Bake for 25 minutes. Let cool before serving.

Tip: You can store these, tightly sealed, at room temperature for up to one week. They are also a delicious garnish for salads, smoothies, or plain yogurt for a tasty breakfast.

Per Serving: Calories: 157; Total fat: 12g; Saturated fat: 2g; Cholesterol: 0mg; Carbohydrates: 6g; Fiber: 2.5g; Protein: 6g

Homemade Applesauce

Grain-Free, Sugar-Free, Vegan

Serves 4 • **Prep time:** 10 minutes • **Cook time:** 40 minutes

There's no particular trick to making good applesauce; you can cook any type of peeled and chopped apples in a little bit of water and you've got a sauce. However, you can boost flavor (and nutrition) by adding spices to the sauce, which is what I've done here. Try this on pancakes, mixed with plain yogurt, or on its own as a delicious snack.

6 apples, peeled, cored, and chopped

1 tablespoon freshly squeezed lemon juice

½ cup water

½ teaspoon Pumpkin Pie Spice Blend (page 131)

1 tablespoon freshly grated ginger

1. In a large pot, toss together the apples, lemon juice, water, Pumpkin Pie Spice Blend, and ginger and bring to a boil over medium-high heat. Lower the heat to medium-low and cook, stirring occasionally, until the apples are soft, about 40 minutes.

2. Mash the apples with a potato masher or blend with an immersion blender. For a smoother sauce, cool the mixture and then puree it in a blender.

Tip: Use crisp, sweet-tart apples such as Braeburns or Granny Smith varieties. One way to add flavor is by using a few different types of apples, which will create complexity and vary the texture of the sauce.

Per Serving: Calories: 144; Total fat: 0.5g; Saturated fat: 0g; Cholesterol: 0mg; Carbohydrates: 38g; Fiber: 6.5g; Protein: 1g

Cocoa and Cranberry Energy Balls

Makes 12 energy balls • **Prep time:** 10 minutes, plus 4 hours to chill

Almond butter makes a creamy base for these delicious low-sugar energy balls. Make as large a batch as you like, place them on a baking sheet, and put them in the freezer. When they are frozen, transfer them to a zip-top plastic bag and store in the freezer for up to six months. Enjoy them any time you want a high-energy snack filled with anti-inflammatory goodness.

½ cup unsweetened almond butter

2 tablespoons honey

2 tablespoons unsweetened cocoa powder

¾ cup old-fashioned oats

¼ teaspoon ground cinnamon

Pinch sea salt

1 tablespoon hot water

¼ teaspoon ground ginger

¼ cup dried cranberries

1. In a large bowl, combine the almond butter, honey, cocoa powder, oats, cinnamon, salt, hot water, and ginger and mix well.

2. Fold in the dried cranberries until combined.

3. Roll the mixture into 12 balls, place them on a plate and cover with plastic wrap, and refrigerate for at least 4 hours.

Tip: Adjust the sweetness to your own taste by using up to 1 tablespoon of additional honey. You can also use maple syrup in place of the honey for a richer flavor.

Per Serving (1 energy ball): Calories: 103; Total fat: 6g; Saturated fat: 1g; Cholesterol: 0mg; Carbohydrates: 11g; Fiber: 2.5g; Protein: 3g

Berries with Honeyed Green Tea Yogurt Sauce

Grain-Free

Serves 4 • **Prep time:** 10 minutes

Green tea is a known metabolism booster and makes an appearance in this simple berry dish, which is both a delicious snack and an equally delicious dessert. If you can't find green tea powder or matcha powder, which is often found in the coffee and tea aisle of the grocery store, it is available online, and it's worth keeping on hand as a valuable addition to a metabolism-boosting kitchen. Of course, you can also omit the tea if you wish, and this dish will still taste great.

½ cup plain nonfat Greek yogurt

2 tablespoons honey

1 tablespoon freshly grated ginger

Juice of ½ orange

½ teaspoon green tea powder

4 cups fresh mixed berries

1. In a large bowl, whisk together the yogurt, honey, ginger, orange juice, and green tea powder.

2. Add the berries and stir until combined. Serve immediately.

Tip: Boost the antioxidant power of this dish by replacing ½ cup of the berries with ½ cup of pomegranate arils (seeds), which you can find in the produce section of many grocery stores.

Per Serving: Calories: 119; Total fat: 0g; Saturated fat: 0g; Cholesterol: 1mg; Carbohydrates: 26g; Fiber: 5g; Protein: 4g

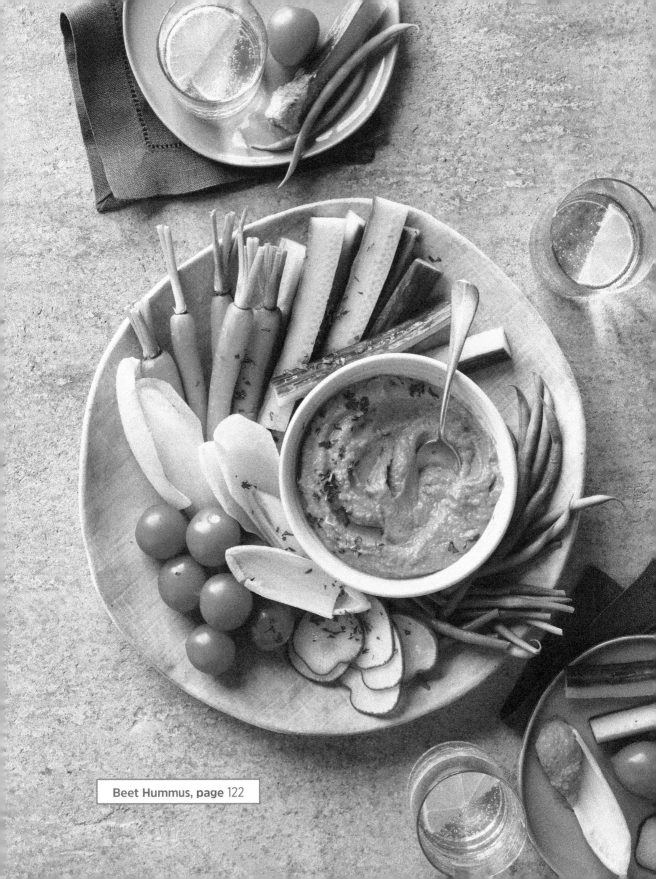

Beet Hummus, page 122

CHAPTER 7

STAPLES

Beet Hummus

Grain-Free, Sugar-Free, Vegan

Makes 2 cups • **Prep time:** 5 minutes

This vividly colored hummus is incredibly good as a dip, and it's delicious in Hummus Deviled Eggs (page 112). It also makes a tasty sandwich spread. The hummus is very versatile; try replacing the canned beets with 1 cup roasted red pepper slices to make a flavorful red pepper hummus.

1 (15.5-ounce) can chickpeas, drained and rinsed

1 cup canned sliced beets, drained

2 tablespoons extra-virgin olive oil

Juice of 1 lemon

2 tablespoons tahini

2 garlic cloves, minced

¼ teaspoon sea salt

In a blender, combine the chickpeas, beets, oil, lemon juice, tahini, garlic, and salt and blend until smooth. Serve immediately or store in an airtight container in the refrigerator for up to five days.

Tip: If you prefer a stronger sesame flavor, you can add up to ¼ cup of tahini to this hummus. For a bit of heat, add up to ¼ teaspoon of cayenne or a dash of chili oil.

Per Serving (¼ cup): Calories: 109; Total fat: 6g; Saturated fat: 1g; Cholesterol: 0mg; Carbohydrates: 11g; Fiber: 3g; Protein: 3g

Spicy Secret Sauce

Grain-Free, Sugar-Free

Makes ¾ cup • **Prep time:** 5 minutes

Every burger and sandwich could be enhanced with a delicious secret sauce like this one. Use it in place of mayonnaise and other condiments for a healthier and still flavorful substitute. It will keep in the refrigerator for up to one week.

½ cup plain nonfat Greek yogurt or plain nondairy yogurt

1 garlic clove, minced

½ teaspoon sugar-free hot sauce

½ teaspoon reduced-sodium soy sauce

2 tablespoons capers, drained, rinsed, and chopped

2 tablespoons chopped fresh chives

In a small bowl, mix the yogurt, garlic, hot sauce, soy sauce, capers, and chives. Taste and add more hot sauce if desired. Use immediately or store in an airtight container in the refrigerator.

Tip: Chili oil also works well to add some heat to this sauce if you can't find sugar-free hot sauce. Add up to ½ teaspoon of chili oil.

Per Serving (2 tablespoons): Calories: 12; Total fat: 0g; Saturated fat: 0g; Cholesterol: 1mg; Carbohydrates: 1g; Fiber: 0g; Protein: 2g

Pico de Gallo

Grain-Free, Sugar-Free, Vegan

Makes 2 cups • **Prep time:** 10 minutes

Pico de gallo is essentially a fresh salsa made with a base of chopped tomatoes. It has many uses, whether as a dip for vegetables, a garnish for Southwestern foods, or a topping for burgers, omelets, or tacos to give them a bit of extra flavor. This will keep in the refrigerator for about four days.

2 large tomatoes, seeds removed, chopped

½ jalapeño, stemmed, seeded, and chopped

½ red onion, finely chopped

1 garlic clove, minced

Juice of 1 lime

¼ cup chopped fresh cilantro

In a small bowl, mix the tomatoes, jalapeño, onion, garlic, lime juice, and cilantro. Use immediately or store in an airtight container in the refrigerator.

Tip: Try making this when tomatoes are in season. Fresh heirloom tomatoes provide the best punch of tomato flavor.

Per Serving (¼ cup): Calories: 13; Total fat: 0g; Saturated fat: 0g; Cholesterol: 0mg; Carbohydrates: 3g; Fiber: 0.5g; Protein: 0g

Buttermilk Ranch Dressing

Grain-Free, Sugar-Free, Vegan

Makes ¾ cup • **Prep time:** 5 minutes

This is a vegan version of buttermilk ranch dressing, so anyone can enjoy it regardless of dietary restrictions. It will keep well in the refrigerator for up to a week, but it always tastes best when you mix up a fresh batch.

¼ cup unsweetened plain nondairy milk (oat milk works particularly well)

3 tablespoons unsweetened plain nondairy yogurt (or silken tofu that has been pureed in a blender)

1 tablespoon apple cider vinegar

2 garlic cloves, minced

1 tablespoon chopped fresh dill

1 teaspoon finely minced shallot

1 tablespoon chopped fresh chives

¼ teaspoon sea salt

¼ teaspoon freshly ground black pepper

In a blender, combine the nondairy milk, nondairy yogurt, vinegar, garlic, dill, shallot, chives, salt, and black pepper and blend until smooth. Use immediately or transfer to an airtight container and store in the refrigerator for up to seven days.

Tip: If you do consume dairy products, you can replace the nondairy milk with low-fat buttermilk and replace the nondairy yogurt with ¼ cup plain Greek yogurt. Omit the apple cider vinegar.

Per Serving (2 tablespoons): Calories: 12; Total fat: 0.5g; Saturated fat: 0g; Cholesterol: 0mg; Carbohydrates: 2g; Fiber: 0.5g; Protein: 0g

Cilantro-Lime Dressing

Grain-Free, Sugar-Free, Vegan

Makes ¾ cup • **Prep time:** 10 minutes

Whether you use it for salads or as a marinade for poultry or fish, this fresh-tasting, pleasantly acidic dressing is sure to enhance the flavors of anything you try it with. It's also extremely versatile, as cilantro and lime flavors work well in both Southeast Asian cuisines and Southwestern or Tex-Mex foods.

¼ cup avocado oil

¼ cup freshly squeezed lime juice

2 garlic cloves, minced

1 tablespoon minced shallot

½ teaspoon Dijon mustard or Chinese hot mustard

¼ cup chopped fresh cilantro

¼ teaspoon sea salt

In a small bowl, combine the oil, lime juice, garlic, shallot, mustard, cilantro, and salt and whisk until blended. Use immediately or store in an airtight container in the refrigerator for up to five days.

Tip: Keep this dressing stored in a jar with a tight-fitting lid and shake it up to remix just before using.

Per Serving (2 tablespoons): Calories: 88; Total fat: 9.5g; Saturated fat: 1g; Cholesterol: 0mg; Carbohydrates: 1g; Fiber: 0g; Protein: 0g

Honey-Mustard Dressing

Grain-Free

Makes ¾ cup • **Prep time:** 5 minutes

This recipe isn't vegan, because it contains honey, but if you are vegan, you can replace the honey with stevia or a similar sweetener without adding extra sugar. This works both as a marinade and as a salad dressing, so it's super versatile.

¼ cup apple cider vinegar

¼ cup Dijon mustard

2 tablespoons honey

½ teaspoon sea salt

2 tablespoons extra-virgin olive oil

In a small bowl, whisk together the vinegar, mustard, honey, salt, and oil until well blended. Use immediately or store in an airtight container in the refrigerator for up to five days. Whisk again just before using.

Tip: For extra flavor, add up to 2 tablespoons of chopped fresh tarragon (or 1 teaspoon dried), which adds a lovely and delicate anise flavor.

Per Serving (2 tablespoons): Calories: 71; Total fat: 4.5g; Saturated fat: 0.5g; Cholesterol: 0mg; Carbohydrates: 6g; Fiber: 0g; Protein: 0g

Ginger-Lime Marinade

Grain-Free, Sugar-Free, Vegan

Makes ½ cup • **Prep time:** 10 minutes

This marinade is good on fish and poultry, but it also serves as a salad or coleslaw dressing in a pinch. It's acidic and aromatic with lots of delicious metabolism-boosting ginger. This will keep in the refrigerator for up to one week.

2 tablespoons avocado oil

¼ cup freshly squeezed lime juice

1 tablespoon reduced-sodium soy sauce

½ teaspoon Chinese hot mustard powder

½ teaspoon sesame oil

1 tablespoon grated ginger

In a small bowl, combine the avocado oil, lime juice, soy sauce, mustard powder, sesame oil, and ginger and whisk until blended. Use immediately or store in an airtight container in the refrigerator.

Per Serving (2 tablespoons): Calories: 74; Total fat: 7.5g; Saturated fat: 1g; Cholesterol: 0mg; Carbohydrates: 2g; Fiber: 0g; Protein: 0g

Citrus-Soy Marinade

Grain-Free, Sugar-Free, Vegan

Makes a generous ¾ cup • **Prep time:** 10 minutes

This marinade is especially delicious with salmon and it also adds flavor to stir-fries. Mix it with plain nonfat yogurt for a creamy spread.

2 tablespoons avocado oil

½ cup freshly squeezed orange juice

1 tablespoon reduced-sodium soy sauce

1 tablespoon freshly squeezed lime juice

1 tablespoon freshly squeezed lemon juice

In a small bowl, combine the oil, orange juice, soy sauce, lime juice, and lemon juice and whisk until blended. Use immediately or store in an airtight container in the refrigerator for up to five days.

Tip: Pour this marinade into a zip-top plastic bag with pork loin, seal, and let marinate in the refrigerator overnight. Remove the pork loin from the marinade and pat dry. Roast in a 400°F oven for about 20 minutes, or until the pork reaches an internal temperature of 145°F.

Per Serving (2 tablespoons): Calories: 49; Total fat: 4.5g; Saturated fat: 0.5g; Cholesterol: 0mg; Carbohydrates: 2g; Fiber: 0g; Protein: 0g

Vegetable Broth

Grain-Free, Sugar-Free, Vegan

Makes 6 cups • **Prep time:** 10 minutes • **Cook time:** 1 hour

Everybody needs a good broth recipe under their belt. Making your own adds flavor, and it isn't terribly difficult to do. Because you're straining off the vegetables and only keeping the broth, you don't even need to take much time peeling or chopping. This broth is made without salt so when you add it to recipes, you can control the salt level depending on what you are making. It can be stored in the freezer for up to six months.

1 onion, halved

2 carrots, washed and cut in half

2 celery stalks, washed and halved

4 garlic cloves, peeled

2 bay leaves

10 peppercorns

2 thyme sprigs

8 cups water

1. In a large pot, combine the onion, carrots, celery, garlic, bay leaves, peppercorns, thyme, and water and bring to a boil over high heat. Lower the heat to medium-low and simmer for 1 hour. Let cool.

2. Strain the broth through a colander set over a large bowl. Discard the solids.

3. Use immediately or store in airtight containers in the freezer for up to six months.

Tip: A great way to minimize food waste in your kitchen is to keep the trimmings from onions (skins and roots), carrots (peels), celery (tops), and herbs in a large zip-top bag in the freezer, and add them along with the other ingredients when you cook the broth. Mushroom ends can also be used to add earthiness to the broth.

Per Serving (1½ cups): Calories: 8; Total fat: 0g; Saturated fat: 0g; Cholesterol: 0mg; Carbohydrates: 2g; Fiber: 0g; Protein: 0g

Pumpkin Pie Spice Blend

Grain-Free, Sugar-Free, Vegan

Makes 3 tablespoons • **Prep time:** 5 minutes

Whether you add this aromatic spice blend to applesauce, sprinkle it over oatmeal, or use it in a smoothie, the delicious combination of metabolism-boosting spices is both fragrant and sweet. You can store it in a zip-top plastic bag (don't forget to label it) in a dark cupboard for up to one year.

2 tablespoons ground cinnamon

1 teaspoon ground nutmeg

2 teaspoons ground ginger

½ teaspoon ground cloves

In a small bowl, stir together the cinnamon, nutmeg, ginger, and cloves. Use immediately or transfer to a zip-top plastic bag for storage.

Tip: Store this in a reused spice jar for easy keeping and dispensing.

Per Serving (1 teaspoon): Calories: 7; Total fat: 0g; Saturated fat: 0g; Cholesterol: 0mg; Carbohydrates: 2g; Fiber: 1g; Protein: 0g

Measurement Conversions

OVEN TEMPERATURES

FAHRENHEIT	CELSIUS (APPROXIMATE)
250°F	120°C
300°F	150°C
325°F	165°C
350°F	180°C
375°F	190°C
400°F	200°C
425°F	220°C
450°F	230°C

VOLUME EQUIVALENTS (LIQUID)

US STANDARD	US STANDARD (OUNCES)	METRIC (APPROXIMATE)
2 tablespoons	1 fl. oz.	30 mL
¼ cup	2 fl. oz.	60 mL
½ cup	4 fl. oz.	120 mL
1 cup	8 fl. oz.	240 mL
1½ cups	12 fl. oz.	355 mL
2 cups or 1 pint	16 fl. oz.	475 mL
4 cups or 1 quart	32 fl. oz.	1 L
1 gallon	128 fl. oz.	4 L

WEIGHT EQUIVALENTS

US STANDARD	METRIC (APPROXIMATE)
½ ounce	15 g
1 ounce	30 g
2 ounces	60 g
4 ounces	115 g
8 ounces	225 g
12 ounces	340 g
16 ounces or 1 pound	455 g

VOLUME EQUIVALENTS (DRY)

US STANDARD	METRIC (APPROXIMATE)
⅛ teaspoon	0.5 mL
¼ teaspoon	1 mL
½ teaspoon	2 mL
¾ teaspoon	4 mL
1 teaspoon	5 mL
1 tablespoon	15 mL
¼ cup	59 mL
⅓ cup	79 mL
½ cup	118 mL
⅔ cup	156 mL
¾ cup	177 mL
1 cup	235 mL
2 cups or 1 pint	475 mL
3 cups	700 mL
4 cups or 1 quart	1 L

Resources

The following resources provide guidelines and information about the functioning and efficiency of metabolism. For more personalized information, seek the advice of a registered dietitian and your doctor.

To understand the food-group targets for your body, visit MyPlate.gov.

To learn more about metabolism and weight loss, visit MayoClinic.org.

To learn what your healthy weight is, visit the "Healthy Weight, Nutrition, and Physical Activity" page at CDC.gov.

References

Johns Hopkins University. "Metabolic Syndrome." Accessed March 9, 2021. HopkinsMedicine.org/health/conditions-and-diseases/metabolic-syndrome.

Murray, Bob, and Christine Rosenbloom. "Fundamentals of Glycogen Metabolism for Coaches and Athletes." *Nutrition Reviews* 76, no. 4 (April 2018): 243–59. DOI.org/10.1093/nutrit/nuy001.

National Institute on Aging. "Research on Intermittent Fasting Shows Health Benefits." February 27, 2020. NIA.NIH.gov/news/research-intermittent-fasting-shows-health-benefits.

US Department of Agriculture and US Department of Health and Human Services. *Dietary Guidelines for Americans, 2020–2025.* 9th ed. December 2020. DietaryGuidelines.gov/sites/default/files/2021-03/Dietary_Guidelines_for_Americans-2020-2025.pdf.

US Department of Health and Human Services. *Physical Activity Guidelines for Americans, 2nd Edition.* Washington, DC: US Department of Health and Human Services, 2018. Health.gov/sites/default/files/2019-09/Physical_Activity_Guidelines_2nd_edition.pdf.

Index

Acknowledgments

I would like to thank the entire production team at Callisto, and I'm especially thankful for the editorial work by Annie Choi. Special thanks to nutrition consultant Karen Frazier for her recipe contributions. I am grateful for the opportunity to reach and help a wider audience become the best versions of themselves.

About the Author

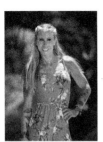

Megan Johnson McCullough is the owner of Every BODY's Fit (EveryBODYsFitOceanside.com) fitness studio in Oceanside, CA. She's an NASM Master Trainer with specializations in fitness nutrition, corrective exercise, senior fitness, drug and alcohol recovery, and AFAA group fitness, and she is a wellness coach, professional natural bodybuilder, and fitness model. This is her sixth published book (see bit.ly /MeganJohnsonMcCullough for a full list). She is happily married to her husband Carl and is the proud mom/owner of two pugs named Steve Nash and Phil Jackson. Currently she is in school working on her doctorate and hopes to help addiction recovery patients using exercise as medicine. She loves to lead by example and give back to the very same community she grew up in through health and fitness.

CPSIA information can be obtained
at www.ICGtesting.com
Printed in the USA
JSHW011233010821
17177JS00001BA/1